PSYCHOLOGY LIBRARY EDITIONS:
PERSONALITY

Volume 9

PERSONALITY DISORDERS

PERSONALITY DISORDERS

New Symptom-Focused Drug Therapy

S. JOSEPH

Routledge
Taylor & Francis Group
LONDON AND NEW YORK

First published in 1997 by The Haworth Medical Press, Inc.

This edition first published in 2019
by Routledge
2 Park Square, Milton Park, Abingdon, Oxon OX14 4RN

and by Routledge
52 Vanderbilt Avenue, New York, NY 10017

Routledge is an imprint of the Taylor & Francis Group, an informa business

British Library Cataloguing in Publication Data
A catalogue record for this book is available from the British Library

ISBN: 978-0-367-03112-1 (Set)
ISBN: 978-0-429-05756-4 (Set) (ebk)
ISBN: 978-0-367-13646-8 (Volume 9) (hbk)
ISBN: 978-0-429-02774-1 (Volume 9) (ebk)

Publisher's Note
The publisher has gone to great lengths to ensure the quality of this reprint but points out that some imperfections in the original copies may be apparent.

Disclaimer
The publisher has made every effort to trace copyright holders and would welcome correspondence from those they have been unable to trace.

S. Joseph, MD, PhD, MPH

Personality Disorders: New Symptom-Focused Drug Therapy

Pre-publication REVIEW

"In a managed care environment, a book that emphasizes appropriate and practical medication strategies targeting specific symptoms of patients with severe personality disorders is long overdue. This book offers the clinician hope that disabling symptoms can be controlled by medications so that psychotherapeutic approaches can be more effective and efficient. Medication should be considered as a first line treatment of patients with personality disorders and not as a last resort when psychotherapy fails. Most personality disorders are treatable using the combination of medication and psychotherapy, and with new medications available, options for effective treatment have increased exponentially. The availability of new, exciting antidepressant and antipsychotic medications has changed the outlook for treatment of personality disorders. This book promises that the most intractable of psychiatric disorders can be treated with excellent outcomes at reasonable costs."

Steven S. Sharfstein, MD
President, Medical Director, and CEO, Sheppard Pratt Health Systems

Personality Disorders
New Symptom-Focused Drug Therapy

S. Joseph, MD, PhD, MPH

HMP

The Haworth Medical Press
An Imprint of The Haworth Press, Inc.
New York • London

CONTENTS

Foreword **xi**
E. Michael Gutman

Preface **xv**

Acknowledgments **xxi**

PART I: PERSONALITY DISORDERS AND CASE STUDIES

Chapter 1. Personality Disorders: General Clinical Concepts **3**
General Diagnostic and Treatment Concepts 14
Symptom-Focused Treatment: The Medical Model 19
Rational Polypharmacy: Evolution in Psychiatric Drug Therapy 23

Chapter 2. Paranoid Personality Disorder **25**
DSM-IV Criteria and Symptom Correlates 25
Symptom Clusters in Paranoid Personality Disorder with Major Medication Options for the Particular Cluster 27
Specific Treatment Recommendations 34
Clinical Cases 1 to 4 35

Chapter 3. Schizoid Personality Disorder **45**
DSM-IV Criteria and Symptom Correlates 45
Clinical Cases 5 to 8 50

Chapter 4. Schizotypal Personality Disorder **57**
DSM-IV Criteria and Symptom Correlates 57
Clinical Cases 9 to 16 62

Chapter 5. Antisocial Personality Disorder **75**
DSM-IV Criteria and Symptom Correlates 75
Clinical Cases 17 to 19 79

Chapter 6. Borderline Personality Disorder **87**

DSM-IV Criteria and Symptom Correlates 87
Treating and Working with Suicidal Patients 94
Clinical Cases 20 to 30 96

Chapter 7. Histrionic Personality Disorder **123**

DSM-IV Criteria and Symptom Correlates 123
Clinical Case 31 127

Chapter 8. Narcissistic Personality Disorder **131**

DSM-IV Criteria and Symptom Correlates 131
Clinical Cases 32 to 35 135

Chapter 9. Avoidant Personality Disorder **143**

DSM-IV Criteria and Symptom Correlates 143
Clinical Case 36 146

Chapter 10. Dependent Personality Disorder **149**

DSM-IV Criteria and Symptom Correlates 149
Clinical Cases 37 to 40 151

Chapter 11. Obsessive-Compulsive Personality Disorder **157**

DSM-IV Criteria and Symptom Correlates 157
Clinical Cases 41 to 48 162

Chapter 12. Personality Disorder, Not Otherwise Specified **173**

Clinical Case 49 173

Chapter 13. Personality Change Due to a General Medical Condition (Axis I) **175**

Common General Medical Conditions That Can Lead to Personality Change 175
Clinical Case 50 178

PART II: CLINICAL PROFILES OF SELECTED PSYCHIATRIC DRUGS

Chapter 14. Clinical Profiles of Selected New Generation Antidepressants **185**

Bupropion (Wellbutrin) and Bupropion SR (Wellbutrin SR) 185
Fluoxetine (Prozac) 190
Sertraline (Zoloft) 192
Paroxetine (Paxil) 194
Venlafaxine (Effexor) 196
Fluvoxamine (Luvox) 199
Nefazodone (Serzone) 201
Mirtazapine (Remeron) 203
Clomipramine (Anafranil) 206
Naltrexone (Revia, Trexan) 207

Chapter 15. Clinical Profiles of Selected New Generation Antipsychotics **209**

Risperidone (Risperdal) 209
Clozapine (Clozaril) 212
Effective Combinations Involving Clozapine 220
Discontinuation of Clozapine 224
Techniques to Detect or Minimize Serious Clozapine Side Effects 226
Starting Clozapine–To Hospitalize or Not 227
Olanzapine (Zyprexa) 239
Sertindole (Serlect) 246

Appendix A. Alphabetical Listing of Drugs by Generic Names, with U.S. Brand Names **253**

Appendix B. Alphabetical Listing of Drugs by U.S. Brand Names, with Generic Names **257**

Appendix C. Alphabetical Listing of Abbreviations **263**

Bibliography **265**

Index **269**

ABOUT THE AUTHOR

S. Joseph, MD, PhD, MPH, is a board certified psychiatrist and licensed clinical psychologist in Orlando, Florida. He is also certified in Geriatric Psychiatry and Addiction Psychiatry and possesses professional training in clinical hypnosis. He received his Master's degree in Public Health from Harvard University and completed his psychiatric specialization at Thomas Jefferson University Hospital in Philadelphia. Dr. Joseph's educational background spans the North American continent. He completed his medical training at the Universidad de Cuidad Juarez in Mexico, his PhD in clinical psychology at the University of Ottawa in Canada, his clinical clerkship in psychiatry at Massachusetts General Hospital, and part of his public health training at the Massachusetts Institute of Technology. Based on his vast experience as a practitioner of psychiatry and psychology, he believes that medication and psychotherapy are equally important for the optimal psychiatric treatment outcome. His success in managing challenging cases validates this belief. Dr. Joseph is a member of the American Medical Association, the American Psychiatric Association, and the American Psychological Association.

Foreword

Personality disorders are enigmatic. Clinicians the world over search for the Holy Grail of understanding the concept and treatment of the elusive personality disorder category.

Dr. Sonny Joseph unlocks the Gordian Knot of understanding and treating personality disorders. Drug therapy universally prescribed for Axis I clinical disorders, ranging from attention deficit disorders (ADD) to zoophobia, had been a heretofore yet-to-be-discovered "diamond-in-the-rough" treatment approach for personality disorders.

Personality Disorders, with the help of snapshot guidelines from the clinician's diagnostic bible, the APA's *DSM-IV,* describes and defines personality disorders, but also outlines solid, easily understood, easily remembered, easily applied cookbook-recipe treatment formats for personality disorders.

Whether you are: (1) the novice undergraduate; (2) the newly-arrived-to-the-patient-scene physician or therapist; or (3) the sage expert clinician, *Personality Disorders* will add vital diagnostic and treatment skills to your armamentarium. Skills that might take years to learn in the usual hunt-and-peck discovery process can be learned quickly through use of *Personality Disorders*.

To better understand the concept of the personality disorder, I would use this analogy: Compare the clinician to an artist who paints a picture and then puts a frame around it. The artist's goal is to tell a story, put it on canvas, and frame it–analyze, and in a way, diagnose a concept, and give a report of the findings. This is so the viewer will know what the artist knows and feels about the subject. The clinician evaluating a patient with a personality disorder has a similar goal of analyzing, diagnosing, and reporting the findings. The clinician paints a picture and frames the diagnosis. The personality disorder represents a unique and rather complex diagnostic dilemma, and every clinician strives to paint, frame, and correctly diagnose the problem of the personality disorder patient.

The personality disorder is unique in that it is not a clinical disorder, or disease entity. It is an intricate mélange of interwoven personality fabrics, adorned with multiple emotional accoutrements. It represents a collage of diverse and manifold personality traits and patterns forming the very essence of the person's presentation to the world. It walks with that person, *as a shadow*, everywhere and every second of the person's existence. It is that shadow, that *collage*, that the clinician must label. The personality disorder is enigmatic, and the clinician is put to a great test having to put the correct diagnostic label on the particular personality disorder that appears before him or her.

Indeed, it often takes more than one visit to outline and describe the long-term, lifelong continuum of patterns and traits that characterize the personality disorder. In a room of ten clinicians offering a diagnosis on a patient with a personality disorder, you might get ten different personality disorder labels, including "Deferred," or "No Diagnosis on Axis II," or "Personality Disorder NOS."

Clinicians with *good* skill, knowledge, education, expertise, training, teaching (mnemonic is SKEETT), can usually hit on target with a reasonably accurate personality disorder diagnosis. Once the objective is reached and a diagnosis is made, the clinician has shown that he or she has the necessary psychic insight into understanding and analyzing the concept behind the patient's condition. Thus, the clinician has painted and framed the picture.

Dr. Sonny Joseph's *Personality Disorders* presents you with a "magic genie assistant" to analyze the enigmatic personality disorder diagnosis and category. Next, *Personality Disorders* gives you the other half of the story–free! The author gives you a recipe-driven cookbook like the *Merck Manual*, like the *PDR*, like Bob Vila's *This Old House*, like *Outdoorsman's Fix-It Book*, like *Hints from Heloise*. It is the best "How To" or "Fix-It" book I have ever read in the field of psychiatry.

Dr. Joseph takes you on a full ride–from the crack of the starting gun: (1) beginning at Part I, Chapter 1, (Personality Disorders: General Clinical Concepts); (2) through 12 separate personality disorder chapters (three clusters, an NOS, and personality change due to general medical condition); and (3) breaking through and ending at the double finish line ribbon–Part II, Chapters 14 and 15

(New Generation Antidepressants and New Generation Antipsychotics).

Dr. Joseph writes in an easily read fashion and delineates his medication program recipes in a one, two, three style format. He offers the clinician who is evaluating and treating the enigmatic personality disorder and its symptoms an innovative, creative, simple, practical, clinical regimen of medicines that helps to alleviate problem symptoms.

This book is the alpha and omega, the beginning and ending of gaining knowledge about the complex subject of personality disorders. It offers new and compelling insights into making the *correct call* on the personality disorder diagnosis. Don't go to the office without it!

E. Michael Gutman, MD, Fellow A.P.A.
Diplomate, Am. Board of Forensic Psychiatry,
Diplomate, Am. Board of Psychiatry with Added on Qualifications in Forensic Psychiatry;
Past President, Florida Psychiatric Society

Preface

Personality disorders are generally considered difficult to treat at best, and untreatable at worst. In fact, personality disorders represent the closest thing to a "four-letter word" in psychiatry. Experienced mental health clinicians frequently hear personality disorder diagnoses stated with a derogatory connotation. It is no secret that psychiatric nurses, psychiatrists, psychologists, and other mental health specialists approach patients having personality disorders with ambivalence, probably emanating from a sense of frustration and helplessness. For example, statements such as "She's a borderline; he is antisocial; he is narcissistic," etc., are commonly used by mental health professionals. It is as if the patients who have personality disorders are contemptible simply because they have them. Generally, treatment of personality disorders is not considered to be as effective as that of Axis I disorders. Traditionally it is held that long-term, psychodynamically oriented, intensive psychotherapy provides the best chance for successful treatment. Relegation of personality disorders to Axis II has perpetuated the notion that personality disorders are less important, and that they are clinical nuisances to be tolerated by clinicians. Primary care physicians particularly have little practical experience in the diagnosis and management of personality disorders.

This book approaches the treatment of personality disorders as if they are Axis I disorders, i.e., with a constructive medical and biological focus. The book analyzes each of the personality disorders in terms of its component symptoms, which are then individually targeted for treatment using selected pharmacological agents. The author had in the past experienced discomfort and frustration when treating patients with symptoms suggestive of personality disorders. Currently, with the conceptualization of these personality disorders in terms of their component symptoms there is now an option that offers hope, direction, and control to a clinician dealing with even the most difficult of personality disorders.

The recent availability of superior medications such as selective serotonin reuptake inhibitors (SSRIs), olanzapine (Zyprexa), risperidone (Risperdal), and clozapine (Clozaril) has been a major factor in this exciting transformation. Medication strategies and dosages are suggested for each of the symptom components that are characteristic of a personality disorder. Clinical techniques for dealing with symptoms that are currently untreatable are also discussed. For instance, there is no medical treatment for defective conscience, one of the features of antisocial personality disorder; yet, there is fairly effective treatment for anger, hostility, irritability, and impulsivity which can be some of the other symptoms of antisocial personality disorder. In this example, the patient, the family, and/or the referring service could then be advised that while there is currently no medical treatment available for a defective conscience and thus none for consequent behaviors such as lying, stealing, and exploiting and hurting others, that treatment can be directed toward other associated specific symptoms. Most other personality disorders are, to a greater or lesser degree, effectively treatable with the balanced use of different medications that address the component symptoms.

Actual clinical cases are presented for all of the personality disorders in order to illustrate the practical applications of the clinical techniques outlined in the book. Most literature to date does not present personality disorders with a detailed focus on the symptoms or with focus on practical pharmacological recommendations. Various clinical presentations discuss the treatable symptoms, including specific medication and dosage recommendations. This emphasis on practical and immediate intervention targeting specific symptoms should have particular applicability in a managed care environment. The clinical cases evoke a "hands-on" feeling in physicians and mental health professionals interested in learning a balanced and correct use of psychotropic medications for the treatment of personality disorders.

Cases were chosen to illustrate various diagnostic and treatment issues including the following:

–Symptom analysis
–Symptom-focused treatment
–Rational use of multiple drugs and dosing strategies

–Treatment ranging from simple to complex methods
–Suicide risk
–Outpatient and inpatient treatment
–Treatment failures
–Clinical skills for successful patient management

Patient identity is of course disguised to assure confidentiality. Clinical history, treatment course, medication doses, and treatment outcome are real. An uneven distribution of cases among various personality disorders is manifest, for example, because some of the personality disorders such as obsessive-compulsive personality disorder, schizotypal personality disorder, and borderline personality disorder come to clinical attention with much greater frequency than avoidant or narcissistic personality disorders. Hence, there are more cases of obsessive-compulsive personality disorder, borderline personality disorder, and schizotypal personality disorder than some of the other disorders.

Each of the 50 clinical cases includes at least one case of each of the personality disorders described in *DSM-IV.* The first paragraph of each case summarizes presenting complaints and symptoms derived from the patient interview, collateral history, mental status examination, and in some cases, psychological test results. Since the main themes of the book are symptom-focused treatment and treatment guidelines, detailed historical information and a section on mental status examination are omitted. As patients typically do not describe their symptoms in clinical terms such as paranoia and suspiciousness, labile affect, odd behavior, suicidal ideation, lack of empathy, dissociative episodes, ideas of reference, hypomania, or obsessive-compulsive tendencies unless they have had psychiatric training, these are listed in the patient's history as conclusions arrived at after studying information from the multiple sources previously listed. In many cases the information summarized in the first paragraph of the case histories was obtained after several patient visits over a period of time. In addition, considerable historical and longitudinal information can be and is obtained from the referring therapist. A unique feature of psychiatric evaluation is that patients sometimes do not divulge all of the information during the first visit. They are more forthcoming with information after they feel comfortable with the clinician. This is particularly true for patients with Axis II disorders, which require longitudinal history, and for patients who have sensitive symptoms or a history which includes suicidal and homicidal ideation, or physical and sexual abuse.

Each case concludes with a comment section that discusses diagnostic and/or treatment issues which are directly or indirectly related to key concepts highlighted in the case. Nearly all of the comments have a practical clinical focus. On reading the cases cited in this text, one might falsely conclude that personality disorders are easily treated and managed. However, personality disorder patients continue to be among the most challenging to diagnose, treat, and manage. The cases selected were chosen because of their successful outcome. Many patients with personality disorders do not respond to treatment with this degree of success and some do not respond at all.

Since virtually all of the clinical cases were based on patient files that were active for a fairly extended period of time prior to 1996 when some of the new medications such as olanzapine (Zyprexa), mirtazapine (Remeron), and lamotrigine (Lamictal) were not available, they could not be included in the clinical cases as active medications that the patients were prescribed. Among the new medications, the author is particularly impressed with the performance of the new atypical antipsychotic olanzapine (Zyprexa), introduced in October 1996. Olanzapine and risperidone (Risperdal) are currently the preferred first-line antipsychotics due to their significantly improved side effect profiles compared to traditional antipsychotics. Their clinical profiles including advantages and disadvantages are described in detail in Chapter 15.

Since diagnostic and treatment concepts are discussed at a fairly advanced level, familiarity with basic psychiatric diagnosis and psychotropic medications is expected of the reader. This text is written primarily for practicing psychiatrists, psychiatric residents, and primary care physicians. Other mental health professionals such as clinical psychologists, social workers, counselors, psychiatric nurses, and medical students considering psychiatric specialization should also find the book relevant and useful.

The section on new generation antidepressants (SSRIs), risperidone, olanzapine, sertindole, and clozapine was reproduced from a book with a broader scope written by the author titled, *Symptom-Focused Psychiatric Drug Therapy for Managed Care* (1997), which may be consulted for practical clinical profiles of the other psychotropic medications in current use, their side effects, and the management of side effects. The technique of symptom-focused treatment of personality disorders, medication strategies, and clinical guidelines described in the book are primarily based on the author's cumulative clinical experience, and might represent clinical art and wisdom, rather than scientifically tested and validated facts. The Bibliography lists sources that were consulted to compile factual information in the book.

Psychotherapy is usually necessary for optimal treatment outcome. It is the author's belief that the gains from psychotherapy are not only significantly enhanced but at times made possible only when the patient's symptoms are satisfactorily controlled with medications. Since the text primarily discusses medical/pharmacological management of personality disorders, the benefit of psychotherapeutic approaches is not specifically mentioned with each discussion of a medication treatment. It is understood that psychotherapy has an important role in the comprehensive treatment of all psychiatric disorders including personality disorders.

The clinical cases 4, 11, 13, 25, 26, 27, 28, 29, and 50 were adapted from *Symptom-Focused Psychiatric Drug Therapy for Managed Care*. The sections on new antidepressants and new antipsychotics are also reproduced from the same source. I am grateful to Anne Carney, MD, Mary Randall, RN, Sandra Houston, PhD, Joseph DeLuca, MD, and Pearline Gardberg, PsyD, for reviewing the manuscript and for offering constructive editorial suggestions. Thanks to Nancy Janisz for preparing the manuscript.

S. Joseph, MD, PhD, MPH
Orlando, Florida

Acknowledgments

I would like to individually thank Bill Cohen, publisher, and all the editors and the production staff at The Haworth Press, including Bill Palmer, Patricia M. Brown, Sandy Jones Sickels, Margaret Tatich, Becky Miller-Baum, Peg Marr, Susan Trzeciak Gibson, Lisa J. Franko, Dawn Krisko, Paula Patton, and Donna M. Brooks. I would also like to thank Dr. Michael Gutman and Dr. Steven Sharfstein for their reviews of the book.

PART I: PERSONALITY DISORDERS AND CASE STUDIES

Chapter 1

Personality Disorders: General Clinical Concepts

It is a popular belief among today's mental health community that personality disorders are untreatable except with long-term psychotherapy, and that psychoanalysis, psychoanalytically oriented psychotherapy, and intensive, long-term behavioral restructuring/retraining are the preferred treatment techniques for most personality disorders. With the advent of a variety of new psychopharmacological agents and judicious use of medication combinations, it is the author's belief, based on vast clinical experience, that most of what we now call personality disorders are treatable to varying degrees of success if their component symptoms are deciphered. Once the symptom configuration is understood, the combination of medications that will address specific symptoms can be identified.

Personality disorders are diagnosed under Axis II disorders according to *DSM-IV* and are typically confusing to other medical professionals. There is an implication that personality disorders are permanent or chronic and that anything other than a structural personality change by means of psychoanalytically oriented psychotherapy or psychoanalysis will not be effective. Such a hopeless attitude toward personality disorders was probably justified several years ago, prior to the advent of new classes of psychiatric medications, such as the SSRIs (selective serotonin reuptake inhibitors), atypical antipsychotics, clomipramine, and others yet to be introduced. The prevalent misinformation in the nonpsychiatric community related to personality disorders is facilitated by the relegation of such disorders to Axis II status. No longer valid is the widely held belief that personality disorders for the most part are untreatable; much of what were thought to be immutable personality characteristics and traits are now modifiable with a variety of medications or combinations of medications.

Psychiatric training must now, to a greater degree, be geared toward understanding our patients' dysfunctional thoughts, feelings, perceptions, and behaviors in terms of symptoms mediated by the brain, rather than as syndromes that exist independently of brain chemistry. Human traits and functions such as character, attitudes, conscience, thinking, perception, and emotions are mediated by the brain. This does not invalidate concepts such as soul, spirit, heart, and mind, which have applicability in the world, but serve only to obscure when goals are medical or psychiatric and not philosophical, religious, poetic, or figurative. Clinicians will attest to the commonness of personality changes that are seen after brain injury. This indicates that changes in anatomic brain structure have an impact on personality; thus, it seems a fair extrapolation to conclude that people with no brain injury are dependent on functional brain characteristics that are alterable with medications which act on the different neurotransmitter systems.

It usually takes years of therapeutic work (and considerable expense) for psychoanalysis to have any chance of success, making the process inefficient, given the human life span as well as the competitive psychotherapy marketplace. The careful use of combinations of medications can make an individual personality less symptomatic, the ultimate goal of psychotherapy. The cost and time associated with pharmacotherapy are also expected to be much less when compared to the psychotherapeutic approach, making the pharmacologic approach much more efficient and thereby more immediately beneficial to the patient in resolving symptoms and saving time. However, as I alluded to in the preface, more than symptoms need to be addressed in providing effective care to patients. Psychological conflicts, lack of insight, poor judgment, relationship issues, social deficiencies, and various other psychosocial issues do not respond to medications, but require psychotherapy for optimal intervention. Therefore, the ideal approach in treating psychiatric disorders–including personality disorders–is primary reliance on the use of medications for the treatment of symptoms and the use of psychotherapy for work related to psychosocial issues and conflicts that can cause symptoms or can be caused by symptoms. Treatment using either approach alone is likely to be incomplete and less successful.

If a symptom is ingrained by being present since childhood or early adolescence it is described as a trait, and thereby considered a personality characteristic that is fairly resistant to change. Examples are emotional instability, moodiness, obsessiveness, social withdrawal, grandiosity, dependency, exaggerated emotions, suspiciousness, emotional sensitivity, and impulsivity. Every characteristic or symptom probably has its correlate in the brain, with the complexity of the control mechanisms varying depending upon the symptoms. Much of these control mechanisms are not precisely understood at the present time and might be sufficiently complex that they will defy complete characterization.

When disinhibition disrupts the tenuous control due to the effects of alcohol, the results are dramatic and mediated by primary process thinking. For example, consider antisocial personality disorder, generally considered the most untreatable of all personality disorders. Individuals with antisocial personalities are said to have a deficient conscience, impaired morality, and an inability to learn from the negative consequences of their behaviors. Currently, it is believed that concepts such as conscience and morality, which are broad and difficult to define, are primarily cortical functions that are more advanced in humans compared to other animals; one can employ the operational concepts such as internal controls and inhibitions to represent the more abstract concepts of conscience and morality, and thereby make the broader concept less vague and more amenable to interventions. Impairment in learning from experience or consequences, another facet of antisocial personality disorder that probably is a result of yet-unknown functional impairment in the brain, leads to deficiencies in internal controls and in inhibitions. Functional deficiencies in the brain must ultimately have their correlates in the structure composed of billions of neurons and their neurochemical and electrophysiological properties. Functions such as perception, learning, thinking, reasoning, inhibitions, conscience, morality, internal control, identity, affect, and judgment are all controlled by the integrative processes in the brain. Optimal balance of inhibitory and excitatory effects might improve the above functions. In antisocial persons, in whom the inhibitory effects are already weak, a disinhibitory drug such as alcohol or a sedative lifts the inhibitions to an extent that previously inhibited behaviors then find their full expression. Many heinous crimes are actually carried out under the disinhibiting effects of alcohol or drugs in susceptible individuals. Highly inhibited people find alcohol helpful in relieving some of the inhibitions; alcohol is used either deliberately or unintentionally for this purpose. Alcohol can have disinhibiting effects resulting in behavioral correlates, providing strong logic in support of the potential to develop drugs having the opposite or inhibitory effect, which promote secondary-process thinking. Other commonly abused drugs that have more complex effects on the brain (most of them undesirable) exist, for example, marijuana, cocaine, LSD, and various narcotics. (In this context, it is interesting to note that nicotine, which is probably one of the most addictive and the most commonly used drugs, has, for the most part, beneficial effects on the central nervous system but is considered unhealthy primarily because of its hazardous effects on other organ systems, especially the respiratory system.)

Because this work is not a treatise on the neurochemical, neurophysiological, and behavioral effects of alcohol and other centrally acting drugs, the purpose of this discussion is intended to provide a brief illustration of the gross effects of centrally acting drugs on behavior. Obviously, the relationship between alcohol and behavior mediated by the brain is highly complex.

Clinical experience leads me to conclude that alcohol or other drugs do not alone cause people to engage in criminal behavior, but that alcohol and other centrally acting drugs have the potential to uncover predispositions in susceptible individuals. The legal argument that alcohol or other prescription or nonprescription drugs make people commit crime may be legally acceptable and therefore might be an appropriate legal defense, but it is not psychiatrically valid or acceptable. Such an argument should not be accepted by a clinician as the sole justification for criminal conduct. A similar but quite distinct scenario would be that of criminal conduct in the context of a true delirium, which can be induced by drugs or various illnesses. For example, the medical determination would be a major factor in a case of a fatal hit-and-run auto accident if delirium obscured the person's very awareness of the victim.

It is clear that our behavior, thoughts, affect, and cognitive processes–even if their patterns are originated in childhood, adolescence–or early adulthood, and are pervasive and stable over time, are controlled by the brain. Thus, if personality is controlled by the brain, interventions that affect brain function have the potential to modify what we describe as personality. Would it not be beneficial to millions (patients and those they affect as well) if there were specific drugs or drug combination therapies that would effectively improve personality characteristics? Clinical experience has convinced me that most personality disorders can at least partially be treated and improved with medication.

In order to successfully treat personality disorders, gross descriptions are useful only in guiding us toward the treatable components. One needs to carefully and systematically elicit and determine individual combinations of symptoms that are present. The goal of psychopharmacologic treatment is to eliminate symptoms that are defined as dysfunctional behaviors, attitudes, perceptions, thoughts, and affects by modifying neurochemical processes in the brain. General diagnostic terms are useful stereotypes, important for communication among professionals, but they lack specificity, making them incapable of determining therapy for individual patients. In order to choose a medication or combination of medications, the most important task is to identify all of the component symptoms the patient is experiencing.

One problem with most personality disorder patients is that it is nearly impossible to get this information from them. In many cases, (1) patients are not cognizant of dysfunctional symptoms; (2) they have forgotten the behaviors; (3) they minimize or deny the symptoms; or (4) since they have had these characteristics or symptoms for so long, they believe that they are part of their inborn personality and therefore are normal or untreatable.

Information from a significant other is beneficial in getting a complete list of symptoms. In the majority of cases, descriptions from a close family member or from someone who knows the patient well are more revealing and can be more valuable than information obtained from the patient. For this reason, when a patient is seen for psychiatric evaluation, it is always helpful to have collateral information from another person who knows the patient well. For example, truly paranoid patients do not have the insight to admit that they are paranoid. When they present to the clinician, typically under coercion, their complaints are likely to be anxiety, depressed mood, insomnia, etc. The benefit of obtaining collateral information from a significant other is not limited to the initial psychiatric evaluation, because collateral input is also helpful during subsequent visits, since the physician gets important additional feedback regarding the behavior of the patient.

It is a common observation that the subtle improvement due to medication during the first several weeks is not perceptible to the patient, but is noticed by others. This is especially true of adolescents who are not very revealing during the initial visits, especially if they have paranoid or antisocial tendencies or personality disorder symptoms. I have seen numerous cases of adolescent patients whose parents complained that the physician who saw the patient previously neither obtained information from them nor gave any feedback. I presume this approach is practiced by clinicians for the desirable purpose of establishing and maintaining therapeutic alliance, rapport, and trust between the clinician and the adolescent patient. However, in a symptom-focused intervention, rapport should not be sought at the expense of obtaining detailed, specific, and thorough clinical information. My experience in treating adolescents is that when the patient realizes that a thorough clinical evaluation, with the help of direct information from the patient and collateral information from as many sources as possible has been performed, rapport will usually follow. The therapeutic alliance is strengthened further by the adolescent's awareness that the clinician is not allowing manipulation of the circumstances. Any therapeutic alliance based on misleading or incomplete information is fragile. If a patient is not giving answers, or gives evasive answers, it is important for the clinician to turn to the parent or significant other and obtain as much history as possible, make an assessment, and suggest treatment based on the information obtained. Rapport and cooperation will follow spontaneously in most cases. These clinical principles are applicable to adults as well, particularly in dealing with personality disorder symptoms and antisocial or severely disordered patients. Because most of these patients come to the clinician as a result of pressure from the family, spouse, employer, lawyer, or court, it is not unusual to hear statements such as "I have been like this all my life," implying that the behavior is normal and that treatment is not needed. It is easier to recognize the irrationality when, for example, a hypertensive individual makes the same statement regarding his/her hypertension. Family members also at times reflect the same thinking in statements such as "He/she has always been like this," or "We are now used to his/her habits." It is the clinician's responsibility to educate both patients and families that even long-standing dysfunctional behavior can be satisfactorily improved by clinical intervention.

For most personality disorders, symptoms can be improved using psychotherapy, medications, and legal interventions. The ideal treatment technique is a combination of judicious use of medication, and psychotherapy, which can take various forms such as behavior therapy, cognitive therapy, group therapy, and psychoanalysis.

My primary objective of this book is to describe in detail how the medication component of treatment can help, and to illustrate how medications can be used in the effective treatment of personality disorder symptoms. The emphasis on medication treatment is not intended to imply that pharmacologic treatment is all that is necessary to help patients. All patients will benefit from psychotherapeutic intervention to some degree; it is highly recommended. However, medications are extremely beneficial, even for patients who pursue psychoanalysis. Based on psychological, physiological, and medical principles, as well as the results in my clinical practice, my opinion is that patients are able to benefit more from psychotherapeutic intervention, including psychoanalysis, when their symptoms are improved with medication.

One potential problem associated with medication intervention is that when some patients achieve significant relief from symptoms, they are then not motivated to continue treatment, including psychotherapy. If patients believe that their improvement is attributable to psychotherapy, they are likely to stop medication and vice versa. Since improvement with medication is initially more obvious than the effects of psychotherapy, which typically takes more effort and more time, it is reasonable to expect that if the medication is effective, the drive to pursue psychotherapy will be diminished. There are, in fact, numerous case examples in which patients decided to discontinue psychotherapy after they had achieved significant improvement from medication. It can be deduced that distress creates the main drive to seek or to continue a treatment. If medication is used to ameliorate the distress, the drive to pursue psychotherapy decreases fairly rapidly. If psychotherapy is used as the sole treatment modality, the drive to continue treatment (psychotherapy) is likely to remain for a longer period of time compared to the pharmacologic approach, because psychotherapy takes more effort and time to produce results in most cases.

There are some qualitative differences by which the two different therapeutic approaches attempt to achieve symptom resolution. A pharmacologic approach primarily attempts to treat symptoms fairly directly, just as antibiotics treat a bacterial infection, or as aspirin treats pain or fever, without much emphasis on attempting to alter factors that may have precipitated the symptoms or illness, such as (continuing the medical example) poor hygiene, exposure to others with the illness, increased stress, and overwork. Once an illness becomes acute, it is not effective to try to use preventive methods to treat the acute phase of the illness. Additionally, if symptoms are not treated fairly rapidly, they can create other complications, such as an untreated fever potentially causing dehydration, weakness, seizures, and delirium.

After the acute illness is brought under control, preventive techniques are important to forestall further episodes. Psychotherapy improves symptoms more in a longitudinal sense by (1) helping people resolve intrapersonal, interpersonal, or other conflicts; (2) helping people to understand themselves, leading to greater emotional control; and (3) helping people to manage stress by teaching various coping mechanisms. These psychotherapeutic benefits might gradually improve symptoms in a patient with an acute illness (as long as the patient does not deteriorate into a crisis state), and at least theoretically, prevent symptoms from occurring in the future. Psychoanalysis historically attempts to restructure a person's personality dynamics, thereby attempting to change the personality in a more functional and healthy direction, making psychoanalysis much more ambitious and comprehensive. The ultimate goal of structural or functional change in personality by means of psychoanalysis or by other techniques is to treat distressing symptoms. Without symptom resolution, structural or any other change in personality has no value to the patient. The eventual purpose of all treatments ideally is to not only improve distressing symptoms, but also to prevent symptoms from emerging in the future. People do not seek treatment simply for the sake of treatment, whether pharmacological or psychological. Treatment is sought when patients are in distress or are symptomatic.

Psychoanalysis, while comprehensive in its goal, is beyond the reach of the majority of patients, especially given the current emphasis on brief interventions that favor medication use. Since there are no qualitative differences between the brains of patients who pursue medication treatment compared to those who seek psychotherapy, and since the brain is controlled by the same neurochemical processes, an adjunctive medication is theoretically beneficial to even those who are in psychoanalysis (which could be considered the ultimate form of psychotherapy and which traditionally does not favor medication). The reason for discussing this topic at length is to emphasize to clinicians that the polarized and concrete thinking held by many traditional psychotherapists has no basis in neurochemistry or in actual clinical experience.

The advent in the early 1990s of the medications that have an improved side-effect profile, has made it virtually imperative that clinicians consider medication treatment for every patient presenting with symptoms while providing psychotherapy that can be universally beneficial. The advantage of combining medication and psychotherapy is that symptom resolution is much more efficient and the chances of relapse are less, compared to either technique being used alone. Because of inherent characteristics, differences in onset of action between the pharmacological and psychological techniques occur, with pharmacological techniques relieving symptoms faster than psychological intervention. Based on these clinical observations, it is suggested that medication be started with or prior to the initiation of psychotherapy, and not as a last resort. In view of the improved safety and efficacy of recently available medications, to not consider therapy with medication for a patient might, in the near future, be suggestive of substandard practice just as not considering psychotherapy for a patient could be considered suboptimal treatment. Given the relatively immediate benefits of medications in rapidly relieving symptoms, there may be some primacy favoring medication intervention in the initial phase of treatment.

The greater efficacy of medication during the initial phase of treatment does not make medication or psychotherapy more or less important in the overall course of treatment, except that differential importance can be attributed at various phases of treatment, and in different diagnoses. To give an extreme example, a patient who is floridly psychotic would immediately need emergency medication management rather than psychotherapy, but would eventually benefit from a combination of maintenance medication and psychotherapy to obtain optimal improvement. Obviously, there is the rare patient who does well on medication alone, and the rare patient who does well on psychotherapy alone, but the greater majority of patients would maximally benefit from an optimal combination of medication and psychotherapy, with individual variations as noted above.

Practical considerations may prevent a particular patient from receiving optimal treatment. For example, medication side effects in a highly medication-sensitive patient, concurrent medications or medical problems interacting harmfully with psychopharmacologic agents, costs, time demands, or poor compliance interfering with psychotherapy can dictate treatment options. Nevertheless, the generic statements regarding the synergistic benefits of combinations of pharmacotherapy and psychotherapy are still valid.

If a characteristic is long-standing and is expressed in the maturing years, that is–in and of itself–a strong reason to suspect that the characteristic in question is primarily constitutional and therefore biologically mediated, making it amenable to biological intervention. In the case of personality disorders, which are characterized by chronic but dysfunctional traits (or symptoms), it makes sense to attempt to treat them as one would treat any symptom that clearly has a physical basis. For some reason, a myth has been perpetuated that long-standing symptoms, as those seen in personality disorders, are not amenable to biological techniques. Therefore, many psychiatrists and physicians do not treat personality disorders with medications. Yet similar symptoms precipitated by psychosocial stressors are routinely treated with medications. From a purely logical standpoint, if any symptoms are likely to be responsive to biological approaches, they would be the personality disorder symptoms (due to their constitutional origins), perhaps even more so than symptoms precipitated by psychosocial stressors. All symptoms, if they cause dysfunction, should be treated using whatever approach is most efficient and most effective.

There is a sense of defeatism among mental health clinicians and psychiatric nursing staff dealing with personality disorder patients. Any clinician who treats psychiatric patients in an inpatient setting knows that patients who are hostile, angry, pessimistic, needy, intrusive, regressed, and complaining are described as having a personality disorder. Similarly, any complicated or difficult patient is also labeled as manifesting a personality disorder. The dysfunctional attitudes and behavior of patients with personality disorders are branded as resistant to improvement; therefore, frequently such behavior is not a focus of treatment. The continued relegation of personality disorders to Axis II status in the *DSM-IV*, besides confusing to nonpsychiatric medical specialists, has not helped to dispel the myth that these disorders are difficult to treat at best and to be avoided at worst. The opinion espoused in this book, based on extensive clinical experience, is that most personality disorders are treatable using a combination of medication and psychotherapy, with judicious use of medication playing an increasingly more important role as a greater range of medication options becomes available. The time has come to treat most Axis II disorders as aggressively and as systematically as the Axis I disorders.

Clinical experience suggests that even some of the symptoms comprising the most untreatable of all personality disorders, namely antisocial personality disorder, can be improved with medications. The possible symptom correlates of each personality disorder listed in *DSM-IV* will be discussed, and specific medication combinations including approximate dosages will be suggested. It is understood that psychotherapy is beneficial to most patients receiving psychiatric medications. This can be assumed in the discussion of each of the personality disorders. The focus of the remainder of the text will be on the identification of symptoms and their medication management.

The central theme of this book is to promote diligent conceptualization and identification of symptom correlates of personality characteristics, regardless of the age at which the characteristics appeared and regardless of whether they are typical of the person's long-term functioning. A personality disorder consists of dysfunctional psychological or behavioral patterns that are enduring, pervasive, inflexible, and distressing. Does this mean that these behaviors are not treatable or should not be treated? To give an example from one nonpsychiatric medical specialty, Would a physical disability go untreated simply because the handicap has been present since birth? The disability would be treated at the time it is discovered if intervention is available, or when intervention becomes available in the future. Until five to six years ago, medication intervention options for personality disorders were limited. The recent availability of exciting new medications has changed this outlook. The aim of this clinical manual is to encourage physicians, psychiatrists, and other clinicians to offer modern medication treatments to improve the lives of our patients suffering from personality disorders.

DSM-IV categorizes personality disorders into three clusters, cluster A, B, and C. Cluster A includes paranoid, schizoid, and schizotypal personality disorders. Cluster B consists of antisocial, borderline, narcissistic, and histrionic personality disorders. Cluster C includes avoidant, dependent, and obsessive-compulsive personality disorders.

GENERAL DIAGNOSTIC AND TREATMENT CONCEPTS

The general diagnostic criteria for a personality disorder according to *DSM-IV* are as follows:*

1. *A pattern of thoughts, attitudes, and behavior that are dysfunctional, pervasive, and abnormal exists, as manifested in at least two of the following areas:*
   a. *Cognitive*
   b. *Affective*
   c. *Interpersonal*
   d. *Impulse Control*

2. *The pattern is evident by adolescence or early adulthood, and is stable and enduring.*

3. *The personality pattern is neither due to another mental disorder, nor due to illicit drugs, medications, or a general medical condition.*

---

*Reprinted with permission from the *Diagnostic and Statistical Manual of Mental Disorders,* Fourth Edition. Copyright 1994 American Psychiatric Association.

A review of the major areas of abnormality manifested in personality disorders shows that these are the same areas that are disturbed in various Axis I disorders. For example, psychosis primarily affects cognitive areas and secondarily impairs affective and interpersonal areas, mania affects all of these areas, and Attention Deficit Disorder primarily affects cognition and impulse control. The differences are in the typical age of onset, chronicity, severity, and pervasiveness. Each of these dimensions is briefly discussed below.

Age of Onset

Symptoms of personality disorders typically emerge during adolescence and early adulthood. Patients with some personality disorders such as antisocial personality disorder and borderline personality disorder come to clinical attention relatively early, due to disruptive manifestations. In the case of antisocial personality disorder, one of the diagnostic criteria is evidence of the presence of conduct disorder with onset prior to age 15. Conduct disorder (before age 18) and antisocial personality disorder (after age 18) are fairly easily recognized by school psychologists and clinicians. Although their short-term prognosis is poor, early diagnosis enables the school, parents, and social and legal agencies to assist the patient in various ways in an effort to limit the dysfunctional effects of the disorder upon the individual and the society.

The onset of schizophrenia also usually occurs in adolescence and early adulthood. Like the personality disorders, schizophrenia is chronic, enduring, and has pervasive effects. Usual ages of onset of various major disorders are listed in Table 1.1.

Based on age of onset, personality disorders do not present any unique features other than a tendency to manifest the characteristics during adolescence and early adulthood. Table 1.1 shows that there are other major disorders that share the same characteristics. The manifestation of personality disorders fairly early in the life cycle suggests that personality disorders may be more biologically determined than is generally believed. If this is true, pharmacological intervention deserves greater emphasis in the management of personality disorders. If treatment is started early, better results are expected.

TABLE 1.1. Age of Onset of Various Psychiatric Disorders

Disorder	Common Period of Onset
personality disorders	adolescence, early adulthood
schizophrenia	adolescence, early adulthood
schizoaffective disorder	early adulthood, adulthood
major depression	adulthood
dysthymia	adolescence, early adulthood
bipolar disorder	early adulthood, adulthood
attention deficit disorder	childhood

Frequently, personality disorders may not come to clinical attention until early adulthood or later when the symptoms exert their cumulative impact on interpersonal, social, academic, occupational, and other important areas of functioning.

Chronicity

Personality disorders are chronic patterns of maladaptive feelings, thoughts, and behaviors, by definition. Axis I disorders such as schizophrenia, delusional disorders, and dysthymia, among others, are also chronic conditions. Thus, it is clear that personality disorders are not unique in the chronicity factor. Since chronic conditions usually require long-term treatment, it is logical to expect that personality disorders will need long-term treatment for optimal benefit.

Severity

There is marked variation in severity among the different personality disorders. Some patients with Borderline Personality Disorder for example, can present with severe dysfunction that is comparable to some of the most dysfunctional Axis I disorders, i.e., schizophrenia and schizoaffective disorders. However, in general, personality disorders are less acute, less severe, and more equitably comparable to Axis I disorders such as dysthymia, anxiety disorders, eating disorders, attention deficit disorder, and obsessive-compulsive disorder. Personality disorders can present with a spectrum of severity as do Axis I disorders, suggesting that qualitatively, personality disorders and Axis I disorders follow similar biopsychosocial characteristics. The general treatment implication is that less acute disorders may respond to low doses of fewer medications for optimal control. Figure 1.1 illustrates the linear relationship between severity of symptoms and medication dose needed for response. For instance, mild psychotic symptoms respond well to a low dose of an antipsychotic while severe psychosis requires a relatively high dose for adequate response. This general observation is based on clinical experience.

FIGURE 1.1. The Linear Relationship Between the Severity of Symptoms and Medication Dose

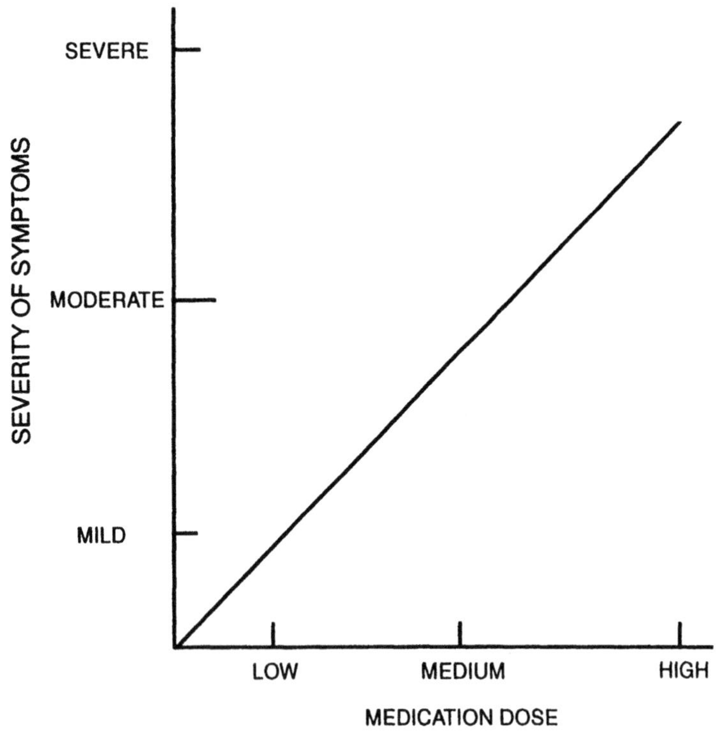

Pervasiveness

Personality disorder affects nearly all aspects of the patient's behavior and relationships. Most Axis I disorders likewise affect a variety of functions in varying degrees. Concerning pervasiveness, personality disorders are more similar than dissimilar to Axis I disorders, which suggest an absence of any qualitative differences.

All of the outlined conclusions imply that the treatment of personality disorders should not be fundamentally or qualitatively different from that of Axis I disorders. Obviously, different disorders within Axis II are variably responsive to treatment due to various factors, such as variations in compliance, potential for insight, and differential response to medications, as is true for Axis I disorders. For instance, factitious disorder, somatoform disorder, and paraphilias, among Axis I disorders, are notoriously difficult to treat.

Several of the personality disorders are more amenable to development of insight and to securing treatment compliance; therefore, they have a better prognosis than other disorders. Table 1.2 shows the prognostic groupings.

TABLE 1.2. Differences in Treatment Compliance Among Personality Disorders

Fair Treatment Compliance (Better Prognosis)	Poor Treatment Compliance (Worse Prognosis)
obsessive-compulsive	antisocial
dependent	paranoid
histrionic	narcissistic
borderline	
schizoid	
avoidant	
schizotypal	

Patients with paranoid, antisocial, schizotypal, schizoid, and narcissistic personality disorders seek psychiatric services typically due to external pressure from a family member, employer, or court system. Once the symptoms are well treated, there is the possibility of developing insight and rapport, which can lead to continued treatment compliance even when external pressures are not sustained. Typically this occurs among paranoid, schizotypal, and schizoid personality disorders, and to some extent in narcissistic personality disorder. The chances of true insight and rapport emerging in antisocial personalities are remote. Although schizoid personalities comply with treatment through a family member's persuasion, treatment effectiveness is modest at best with currently available medication interventions.

SYMPTOM-FOCUSED TREATMENT: THE MEDICAL MODEL

If the physician is able to identify the symptoms that are causing distress to a patient, regardless of the personality disorder diagnosis, treatment should be offered. In some cases, one medication may effectively address multiple symptoms, whereas in other cases, multiple medications are necessary for optimal symptom control. In the former case, a patient with three or four distinct and disparate symptoms can be treated with one medication, whereas in the latter case, a person with three or four different symptoms may need three or four medications from different classes depending upon the specific symptoms. In rare instances multiple medications may be necessary for the optimal control of one symptom. The following simplified hypothetical examples will illustrate this point.

1. A healthy 30-year-old patient presents with depressed mood, obsessive rumination of the fear of dying of cancer, mild compulsive cleaning behavior, anxiety attacks, and anger outbursts. In this example, there are four different target symptoms as follows:

    1. Depressed mood
    2. Obsessive-compulsive features
    3. Anxiety
    4. Anger

All of the above symptoms might effectively be treated with one medication, for instance with one of the serotonergic antidepressants* such as fluoxetine, sertraline, paroxetine, venlafaxine, mirtazapine, and fluvoxamine, or with clomipramine, or with one of the tricyclic antidepressants (TCAs). The author prefers a first trial on serotonergic antidepressants (SSRIs), then clomipramine, and then TCAs, primarily because of the benign side effect profile of SSRIs. The ideal goal is to treat the symptoms using one medication, which is quite possible if the symptoms are as listed above. However, such an economy is not always possible, as will be seen in the next hypothetical case example.

2. A healthy 30-year-old patient presents with symptoms such as depressed mood, frequent nightmares causing sleep disruption, paranoid ideation, and significant mood swings.

   The four different target symptoms are:

   1. Depressed mood
   2. Nightmares
   3. Paranoid ideation
   4. Mood swings

This patient also has four different symptom foci; however, adequate resolution of these four symptoms could require the use of medications from four different classes as follows:

Symptom	Medications
Depression	antidepressant, preferably an SSRI
Nightmares	benzodiazepine at bedtime, or low dose of a TCA at bedtime
Paranoia	low dose of an antipsychotic
Clinically significant mood swings	mood stabilizer

3. A healthy 30-year-old patient presents with hostility. The only target symptom is hostility. This patient could require medications from different classes for the best outcome.

*"Serotonergic antidepressants" is used loosely in this context to include all of the new generation antidepressants such as fluoxetine, sertraline, paroxetine, venlafaxine, fluvoxamine, and mirtazapine. Venlafaxine and mirtazapine have both sertonergic and noradrenergic effects.

Symptom	Medications
Hostility	SSRI and antipsychotics at low doses (risperidone or olanzapine preferred due to favorable side effect profile)

The key concept is global improvement via symptom control, through treatment with effective medication for each symptom identified. The patients' complaints are translated into individual symptoms (no matter how many there might be) that are then targeted for treatment; progress is then followed in an organized and disciplined manner. Drugs that are not effective are eliminated, and drugs that become unnecessary over time are reduced or discontinued. Conversely, a symptom that improves partially may respond to increasing drug doses or addition of other medications as dictated by the clinical problem.

Unfortunately, when dealing with psychiatric problems, many excellent physicians do not think in the same clinically precise manner that they would employ if they were treating a nonpsychiatric illness. Again, a medical example illustrates this idea. A 42-year-old patient presents with symptoms of clear rhinorrhea, dyspnea upon exertion, postprandial bloating, premenstrual cramps, low backache, productive cough, and heartburn. Exam findings indicate a blood pressure of 175/102 and are otherwise consistent with benign etiologies for all of the patient's complaints. Additional history is a five-year history of borderline hypertension, a family history of essential hypertension, and a cyclic history of seasonal allergies, frequently with reactive airways. The diagnoses then are: seasonal allergies with rhinorrhea; allergic asthma; probable lactose intolerance; essential hypertension; premenstrual syndrome; lumbar strain; bronchitis; and gastritis/reflux esophagitis. The primary care physician will have no hesitation in considering several medications from several classes as follows:

Symptom	Medications
Rhinorrhea	antihistamines, decongestants
Asthma	bronchodilators, steroids

Symptom	Medications
Essential hypertension	diuretics, beta blockers (both undesirable with asthma), calcium channel blockers, ACE inhibitors, alpha-2 agonists, peripheral vasodilators, etc (and physical measures)
Lactose intolerance	lactase
Premenstrual cramps	nonsteroidal anti-inflammatory, oral contraceptives, aspirin, acetaminophen
Lumbar strain	nonsteroidal anti-inflammatory
Bronchitis	antibiotics
Gastritis/reflux esophagitis	H_2 blockers, omeprazole, antacids

While this comparison between the medical and psychiatric approaches has its limits (psychiatrists do not generally search for occult diseases as rigorously as medical practitioners look for cancers, for example), it does reinforce the point that when it comes to nonpsychiatric problems, physicians have no difficulty organizing the symptoms and prescribing a medication for each specific target symptom. Returning to the hypothetical case, this patient could be prescribed eight different medications for eight different problems. Fewer than eight medications could be considered suboptimal treatment. Some combinations of medications might be contraindicated, or in another circumstance, one medication will serve for two or more symptoms. It is not at all uncommon to see a medical patient taking three, four, ten, or even more medications from different pharmacologic classes. As in psychiatry, this entire list of medications is not permanent, with medication for acute symptoms being eliminated as soon as the patient's condition allows, with antihypertensives more likely to be a lifelong necessity. Physicians tend to think clearly, logically, and specifically when dealing with nonpsychiatric symptoms. The time has come in psychiatry for psychiatric specialists as well as primary care physicians to apply this same clinical precision on a more general scale, i.e., to use it in the management of psychiatric problems. The management of personality disorders is no exception.

RATIONAL POLYPHARMACY: EVOLUTION IN PSYCHIATRIC DRUG THERAPY

Polypharmacy carries a negative connotation of too many drugs, conflicting drugs, and lack of physician care and attention to the complete drug list so that multiple specialists are together prescribing a mishmash of medications with toxic potential. More precisely, however, the word polypharmacy in its pristine form means "multiple drugs." While the negative connotation indicates too many, the more correct definition–as adhered to in this text–should elicit a positive connotation of only as many drugs as are necessary, each for a specific target symptom, each evaluated individually for efficacy and side effects and adjusted optimally, and each eliminated when no longer necessary.

Some years ago when there were only three or four classes of psychiatric medications available, each with many common side effects and less specific main effects, concurrent use of more than one class of medication was likely to lead to adverse effects. However, in recent years, more and more new psychiatric medications with specific indications and effects have become available, affording use of intelligent drug combinations for optimal symptom control. Inevitable and desirable evolution in psychiatric drug therapy has made it possible to practice rational polypharmacy, which every contemporary psychiatrist must learn to provide the patients with the best care possible in an era of psychopharmacological revolution.

Chapter 2

Paranoid Personality Disorder

The diagnostic criteria for paranoid personality disorder, according to *DSM-IV*, are given below:*

DSM-IV *CRITERIA AND SYMPTOM CORRELATES*

A. A pervasive distrust and suspiciousness of others such that their motives are interpreted as malevolent, beginning by early adulthood and present in a variety of contexts, as indicated by four (or more) of the following:

1. *Suspects, without sufficient basis, that others are exploiting, harming, or deceiving him or her.*
2. *Is preoccupied with unjustified doubts about the loyalty or trustworthiness of friends or associates.*
3. *Is reluctant to confide in others because of unwarranted fear that the information will be used maliciously against him or her.*
4. *Reads hidden demeaning or threatening meanings into benign remarks or events.*
5. *Persistently bears grudges, i.e., is unforgiving of insults, injuries, or slights.*
6. *Perceives attacks on his or her character or reputation that are not apparent to others and is quick to react angrily or to counterattack.*
7. *Has recurrent suspicions, without justification, regarding fidelity of spouse or sexual partner.*

B. Does not occur exclusively during the course of schizophrenia, a mood disorder with psychotic features, or another psychotic dis-

---

*Reprinted with permission from the *Diagnostic and Statistical Manual of Mental Disorders,* Fourth Edition. Copyright 1994 American Psychiatric Association.

order and is not due to the direct physiological effects of a general medical condition.

The approximate symptom correlates for each of the paranoid personality characteristics are listed in Table 2.1.

Obviously, there is considerable overlap in the criteria and therefore in the symptom correlates. The symptoms can be grouped into several distinct categories as explained in the next section. These different categories of symptoms respond to different classes of medications, again with some overlap. For example, obsessional

TABLE 2.1. Symptom Correlates for Paranoid Personality Disorder

DSM-IV **Criteria**	**Possible Symptom Correlates**
1. Suspects, without sufficient basis, that others are exploiting, harming, or deceiving him or her	paranoia
2. Is preoccupied with unjustified doubts about the loyalty or trustworthiness of friends or associates	obsessional features, anxiety, paranoia
3. Is reluctant to confide in others because of unwarranted fear that the information will be used maliciously against him or her	paranoia, vigilance, guardedness, constricted affect, social withdrawal, seclusiveness, social anxiety
4. Reads hidden, demeaning, or threatening meaning into benign remarks or events	mild ideas of reference, excessive emotional sensitivity
5. Persistently bears grudges, is unforgiving of insults, injuries, or slights	anger, extreme sensitivity
6. Perceives attacks on his or her character or reputation that are not apparent to others and is quick to react angrily or to counterattack	mild ideas of reference, anger attacks, irritability, vigilance
7. Has recurrent suspicions, without justification, regarding fidelity of spouse or sexual partner	paranoia

symptoms, dysphoria, anxiety, and anger attacks all respond well to serotonergic drugs. However, for the sake of clarity I will list the distinct treatable symptom correlates and give the corresponding medication classes, as well as specific medication combinations and dosage ranges to achieve optimal symptom resolution.

SYMPTOM CLUSTERS IN PARANOID PERSONALITY DISORDER WITH MAJOR MEDICATION OPTIONS FOR THE PARTICULAR CLUSTER

Paranoia, Mild Ideas of Reference

Example of low dose antipsychotic:

- risperidone (Risperdal) 0.5 mg or 1 mg AM or HS, or olanzapine (Zyprexa) 1.5 to 3.75 mg HS, the author's preferred neuroleptics

Other drugs include the following:

- haloperidol (Haldol) 0.5 to 2 mg HS
- fluphenazine (Prolixin) 0.5 to 2 mg HS
- trifluoperazine (Stelazine) 0.5 to 2 mg HS
- perphenazine (Trilafon) 2 to 4 mg HS
- thiothixene (Navane) 1 to 2 mg HS
- loxapine (Loxitane) 10 to 25 mg HS
- molindone (Moban) 10 to 20 mg HS
- mesoridazine (Serentil) 10 to 25 mg HS
- thioridazine (Mellaril) 10 to 50 mg HS
- chlorpromazine (Thorazine) 10 to 50 mg HS

Success in using neuroleptics for the treatment of low-grade paranoia depends on the dosage. For patient acceptance and to minimize side effects, it is important to start at a very low dose. These dosages are approximately one-tenth to one-fourth of what is used for treating florid paranoia and psychosis. Examples of ranges of neuroleptic dosages are given above. For a given patient, the dosage must be individually tailored, and may be less than or exceed the ranges given. It is preferred that the antipsychotic is given as a one-time dose at bedtime to minimize daytime sedation. The author's clinical experience suggests that antipsychotics are very effective in decreasing the intensity of paranoia, even if it is long-standing and mild. Since paranoid patients are generally very intolerant of side effects, the clinical strategy is to start at homeopathic doses, and as the level of paranoia decreases and the patient becomes comfortable with the medication, to increase the dosage gradually, if needed. In the treatment of paranoid personality disorder, an antipsychotic alone is usually not sufficient for optimal benefit, as outlined above. Other symptoms which are present need to be treated for satisfactory results. Case #1 illustrates this principle.

Obsessional Features

Obsessional, rigid, and concrete thinking are common and characteristic symptoms in paranoid personality disorder (as well as in Axis I delusional disorders). If obsessional symptoms are recognized in paranoid personality disorders, appropriate treatment can be initiated, leading to overall treatment success. The various medications and dosage ranges the author has found beneficial are given here.

- clomipramine (Anafranil) 25 to 225 mg (in divided doses)
- fluoxetine (Prozac) 20 to 80 mg QD
- fluvoxamine (Luvox) 50 to 300 mg QD
- sertraline (Zoloft) 50 to 200 mg QD
- paroxetine (Paxil) 20 to 60 mg QD
- venlafaxine (Effexor) 25 to 125 mg TID

In general, obsessional symptoms require higher dosage ranges of the above medications, as compared to depressive or anxiety symptoms. For example, a dose of clomipramine 75 mg TID or fluoxetine 60 mg QD is frequently needed for resolution of obsessional symptoms in obsessive-compulsive disorder, whereas depressive and anxiety symptoms tend to respond on the average at approximately half the dosage noted above. The unique problem associated with the treatment of obsessional symptoms in paranoid personality disorder is that although the patients will require dosages in the middle to upper dosage range, since they are sensitive to and intolerant of side effects, the initial dosage must be low, with slow dosage increments, in order to allow time for the development of tolerance to the side effects.

Vigilance, Guardedness, and Tension

Vigilance, guardedness, and tension are paranoid manifestations with a predominant anxiety component for which treatment using very low doses of benzodiazepines for a short period of time is beneficial. Such adjunctive treatment, coupled with serotonergic antidepressants and very low doses of antipsychotics, is effective in enabling patients to function better interpersonally. This treatment also enables patients to agree to enter psychotherapy, thereby potentially helping them to gain better insight into their problems. Even uncooperative and unmotivated patients can benefit from treatment and may stay in treatment if they experience a certain level of improvement without side effects, because the improvement in their symptoms gives them an opportunity to acquire some insight and to develop rapport. Paranoid patients have difficulty relaxing even during the therapy session; they are tense, vigilant, and constantly stressed. They do not have the insight to admit to this, prior to treatment. It is the author's belief, confirmed by clinical experience, that paranoia typically leads to secondary symptoms of anxiety, depression, and insomnia, which are often the presenting symptoms, as exemplified by Case #2. Anxiety, which is a universal symptom in paranoid individuals, must be treated adjunctively, preferably using low doses of benzodiazepines for two to three weeks or until the serotonergic antidepressant and low dose antipsychotic have time to exert their optimal effects on the patients' thinking and mood. The key clinical strategy is to start patients on extremely low doses so that sedation or somnolence will not be a side effect. Examples of adjunctive benzodiazepines in paranoid personality disorder follow.

- lorazepam (Ativan) 0.5 mg 1/2 tablet BID-TID
- alprazolam (Xanax) 0.25 mg 1/2 tablet TID-QID
- clonazepam (Klonopin) 0.5 mg 1/2 tablet BID

- diazepam (Valium) 2 mg HS
- chlordiazepoxide (Librium) 5 mg HS

On such low doses, patients are unlikely to experience any significant sedative side effects. As vigilance and guardedness serve a protective psychological function for paranoid individuals, to simply remove these symptoms by the use of benzodiazepines without treating the underlying paranoia and thought disorder is likely to be frightening to these patients; hence, benzodiazepines at low doses should be an adjunctive rather than primary treatment. Clinical experience indicates that satisfactory treatment of the basic paranoid symptoms could relieve the excessive vigilance and guardedness, thereby eventually obviating the need for benzodiazepines.

Anger, Excessive Emotional Sensitivity, and Irritability

All serotonergic antidepressants have excellent efficacy in decreasing anger and in increasing emotional control. Tricyclic antidepressants are also effective. Bupropion is moderately effective, but less so compared to serotonergic medications.

Constricted Affect and Social Withdrawal

These symptoms may represent mild forms of "deficit" or "negative" symptoms. They are likely to respond to low doses of risperidone or olanzapine and, paradoxically, to serotonergic antidepressants and bupropion.

Treatment Strategy

Ideal treatment is a combination of medications followed by addition of supportive psychotherapy with interpersonal and insight components. Regressive or intrusive techniques or excessive focus on insight can be counterproductive. It is clear from the previous discussion that there are various symptom clusters which are preferentially responsive to different medications. For optimal outcome, simultaneous treatment of all of the major symptom clusters may be necessary.

Symptom Cluster	Medication Options
Paranoia	low dose antipsychotics, preferably risperidone or olanzapine
Obsessive features, irritability, sensitivity, anger, social anxiety, dysphoria	antidepressants, particularly serotonergic antidepressants or clomipramine (Anafranil)
Anxiety, vigilance	very low dose benzodiazepines for brief period of time or on a PRN schedule

It is easy to understand and remember the diagnostic criteria for paranoid personality disorder. However, it is difficult to elicit the presence of behaviors suggestive of paranoid personality disorder from the patient directly. Paranoid personality characteristics manifest themselves typically in interpersonal conflicts with close individuals such as spouses, supervisors, colleagues, and relatives, and it is usually at their insistence that the patient reluctantly agrees to come in for a psychiatric evaluation or for counseling. The diagnosis is frequently missed unless the collateral information from significant others is obtained by the clinician. If the true diagnosis is missed, the misdiagnosis commonly made is one of the anxiety or dysthymic disorders, with a prescription for a benzodiazepine or an antidepressant, which will provide some relief, but not optimal relief of symptoms. Hence, it is always helpful to the clinician to get information from collateral sources. It is the author's practice to invite close family members or significant others into the office along with the patient for the first visit, with the opportunity given to the patient to reveal sensitive information either before or after the interview of the family member or significant other. If the patient comes alone for the interview, an attempt should be made to contact collateral sources by phone to get a complete history of the patient's difficulties. If a patient refuses permission for the clinician to contact a collateral source either in person or on the phone without reasonable explanation, one should seriously consider paranoia in the differential and search for other supporting clues. It is not facetious to suggest that clinicians must have a high index of suspicion to diagnose paranoia, especially the mild paranoia present in paranoid personality disorder because almost all paranoid patients are clever in guarding their paranoid traits, more than any other category of patients. They rigorously test the clinician's clinical skills in diagnosis and treatment. Some of the techniques the author has found useful are described in the treatment section. In most other conditions, once the diagnosis is made, treatment simply ensues. In paranoid individuals, both diagnosis and overcoming the patients' resistance to treatment are difficult to accomplish, at best. Case #4 is an example.

Paranoia, guardedness, suspiciousness, etc., are inferences that the clinician makes based on descriptions of behaviors and the clinical observations, patient history, collateral history, and mental status examination. A clinician should not typically ask a patient, "Are you paranoid?" because the answer is likely to be "No." In contrast, other symptoms such as depression, anxiety, phobia, or obsessive-compulsive conduct may be elicited by direct questioning. Once paranoia is diagnosed, the clinician must be tactful and empathetic to get the patient to comply with treatment. Patients with even mild paranoia are unhappy (if not depressed), anxious, tense, frustrated, and unable to relax. They tend to have insomnia, anxiety attacks, and vague physical complaints. This understanding should be conveyed to the patient in an empathetic manner with a statement similar to the following: "It must be such a stress for you to have these thoughts and feelings," or "It must be difficult for you to have peace of mind when you feel this way." Once the presence of paranoia is identified, it is more useful for purposes of communication with the patient to employ phrases such as "anxiety thoughts" or "stressful thoughts" rather than to refer to paranoia, especially in the initial stages of evaluation and treatment. Once the patient improves, he or she may become less guarded when words such as "paranoia" and "suspiciousness" are used. However, the author has found that these words are too emotionally loaded and tend to make patients mount their defenses; hence, a gentle and indirect approach is preferable in dealing with paranoid patients.

Paranoid patients need considerable reassurance and persuasion to accept treatment. The clinician should not engage in a debate regarding their diagnosis or try to reason with them, beyond simply saying that they are under stress, that their life is being affected by these stresses and anxiety thoughts, that simple and effective treatment is available, and that they should make a determined effort to follow the treatment plan. The clinician should anticipate their defenses, such as projection, denial, rationalization, and intellectualization, and attempt to work with the awareness that these defenses may interfere with treatment. Emphasize that the medications are at low doses. Educate the patient about and encourage them to bear with the common and benign side effects such as nausea, heartburn, sexual dysfunction, headaches, slight sedation, tired feeling, and nervousness, almost all of which usually subside over time.

Antipsychotics

The author's first-line antipsychotics are risperidone, which is usually given in doses of 0.5 mg to 2 mg, and olanzapine given in doses of 1.25 to 3.75 mg, if possible as one-time doses at night. Risperidone and olanzapine are preferred because of their favorable side effect profile compared to other antipsychotics and their mild to moderate effect on "negative" or "deficit" symptoms. If risperidone or olanzapine is not tolerated or is not effective, other antipsychotics may be tried. The author's experience suggests that for minimizing side effects and for patient compliance, the starting dosage should be lower than the starting dose recommended by the manufacturer. A starting dose of risperidone 0.5 mg per day is recommended, with increments of 0.5 mg every week, if necessary. Many patients will respond well at 0.5 mg per day. For olanzapine a starting dose of 2.5 mg HS is recommended. Rapid dosage escalation usually leads to side effects and noncompliance.

Antidepressants

In general, SSRIs (selective serotonin reuptake inhibitors) are preferred due to fewer side effects, as compared to TCAs (tricyclic antidepressants) and MAOIs (monoamine oxidase inhibitors). However, clomipramine's anticholinergic property can be of some benefit for a patient who is on high potency antipsychotics such as haloperidol, fluphenazine, trifluoperazine, thiothixene, and perphenazine, as well as risperidone because clomipramine, besides treating the obsessional symptoms frequently found in paranoid patients, can ameliorate possible EPS (extrapyramidal symptoms) induced by the antipsychotics. However, since serotonergic antidepressants have a very favorable side effect profile, clomipramine's anticholinergic property should not be the primary attraction especially if an average or high dosage range of clomipramine is to be used. Besides, the low dosage of antipsychotics employed in the treatment of paranoid personality disorder often cause relatively fewer side effects. This consideration is not applicable if low-potency antipsychotics such as thioridazine, chlorpromazine, and mesoridazine are used. In fact, anticholinergic toxicity can result if high doses of low potency antipsychotics and highly anticholinergic antidepressants are combined, and should be avoided in treatment for everyone, particularly the elderly and children.

Since paranoid individuals are very defensive and sensitive, they are likely to notice even the most benign side effect. They should be educated about and prepared for tolerating possible side effects.

Antianxiety Medications

Low doses of intermediate or fairly short-acting benzodiazepines are preferred. The dosage should be low, to avoid any sedation, which can lead to noncompliance. The dosage should be just enough to take the "edge" off of the anxiety and vigilance, but not make the patient somnolent.

SPECIFIC TREATMENT RECOMMENDATIONS

For optimal treatment of paranoid personality disorder, three different classes of medication are needed in most cases. A low dose antipsychotic and either clomipramine or one of the serotonergic medications are administered on a fairly long-term basis (one to two years). A very low dose of a benzodiazepine is helpful for short-term use, especially in the initial stages of treatment, and then on an "as needed" basis for treatment of episodic anxiety. The addition of comfort medications such as a hypnotic and an appetite stimulant may be useful in individual cases. Examples of maintenance prescriptions for patients with paranoid personality disorder could be as follows:

Patient A

- risperidone 0.5 mg HS
- clomipramine 100 mg HS
- lorazepam 0.25 mg BID-TID (1/2 of a 0.5 mg tablet)

Patient B

- olanzapine 2.5 mg HS
- fluoxetine 20 mg AM (or one of the other serotonergic antidepressants)
- alprazolam 0.125 mg TID (1/2 of a 0.25 tablet)

Patient C

- haloperidol 0.5 mg HS
- paroxetine 20 mg AM
- clonazepam 0.25 mg BID (1/2 of a 0.5 mg tablet)

Patient D

- mesoridazine 25 mg HS
- fluvoxamine 100 mg BID
- lorazepam 0.25 mg BID

If a patient on these medications complains of insomnia and loss of appetite, the addition of doxepin 10 mg or an equivalent TCA at bedtime and, if needed, increasing the dose of benzodiazepine at bedtime will usually help without significant side effects. Cases 1 to 4 discuss practical issues related to the pharmacological treatment of paranoid personality disorders.

CLINICAL CASES 1 to 4

Case #1

Presenting Symptoms: The patient was a 39-year-old female, with complaints of unsocial behavior, mild ideas of reference, suspiciousness, distrust of others, social isolation, excessive emotional sensitivity, and excessive anger. These symptoms had been present since her late teens and were described as being part of her "nature." She was coerced into coming to the psychiatrist's office by her husband who had been extremely frustrated by her attitudes and behavior. The husband was seriously considering divorce when the patient was first seen. She denied drug and alcohol abuse, smoking, and caffeine intake. She also denied previous psychiatric evaluation or treatment. The patient's aunt had paranoid schizophrenia. The patient's medical history was unremarkable.

Axis II Diagnosis: Paranoid personality disorder with schizoid features

Current Treatment: 1. risperidone 0.5 mg HS
2. fluoxetine 10 mg AM

Treatment Course: The patient was initially started on a combination of perphenazine 2 mg and amitriptyline 10 mg (Triavil 2-10) at bedtime and fluoxetine 20 mg AM. She tolerated this combination well for a year, after which mild tremors of the upper extremities and mild involuntary vermiform tongue movements occurred. Triavil was discontinued and she was switched to risperidone 0.5 mg at bedtime, which resulted in regression of the involuntary movements. After about a year of being on fluoxetine 20 mg, the dose was decreased to 10 mg with no significant loss of therapeutic benefits. All of the paranoid symptoms improved significantly. Social withdrawal and lack of interest in social activities continue to persist; however, her husband and other family members are happy with her progress. The patient has acknowledged that she feels better on the medications and has been taking medications regularly without urging by her husband. An attempt to discontinue fluoxetine resulted in increased anger and moodiness. Decreasing the dose of risperidone to 0.25 mg led to the recurrence of paranoid symptoms. The patient is expected to be maintained on the current medications and at the current dose indefinitely. The combination of risperidone 0.5 mg HS and fluoxetine 10 mg AM resulted in remarkable improvement in this patient's quality of interpersonal interactions. The marital feuds that were common prior to starting medication treatment have become rare and less intense.

Comments: Patients, or significant others who bring the patient for a psychiatric evaluation, do not succinctly list the symptoms as poor social skills, mild ideas of reference, suspiciousness, distrust of others, excessive emotional sensitivity, and excessive anger. These are symptom designations that the clinician infers from detailed descriptions of patients' behavior, feelings, and attitudes by the patient and/or significant others in response to inquiries by the clinician. A truly paranoid patient is unlikely to tell the clinician that he or she is paranoid. In fact, they usually deny or become offended if they are directly asked questions regarding their paranoid thinking. When paranoia is severe, it takes only a few seconds of observation or a brief inquiry to diagnose it. However, with paranoid personality disorders, careful review of presenting complaints and, perhaps more important, collateral history from significant others, as well as a high index of suspicion by the clinician are necessary to diagnose paranoia. Such an approach is needed for identifying the presence of most mild symptoms that are typical of most personality disorders. Even after the presence of paranoia in a patient is confirmed, it is best to avoid asking patients directly regarding the status of their paranoia. Clinicians should be able to infer the existence of paranoia from the patient's demeanor, facial expression, behavior, and interpersonal interaction. Questions regarding paranoia may be asked indirectly as follows, if necessary:

- Have those anxiety thoughts lessened?
- Are you still as fearful?
- Are you better able to trust people now?
- Are people treating you better now?
- Are people more friendly to you these days?
- Do you feel more relaxed after starting the medications?

Patients with paranoid personality disorder rarely seek treatment voluntarily. Typically, a family member or employer persuades them to seek help. The adverse consequences of paranoid personality features are primarily manifested in interpersonal contexts. Many marital conflicts, divorce, and family feuds are caused by untreated paranoid personalities. Mild forms of paranoid personality features are almost impossible to diagnose unless the clinician is very vigilant to the presence of underlying paranoia. Moreover, if they present to the clinician in an office, the presenting symptoms usually are anxiety and depression, further obscuring the true diagnosis. Often antidepressant and/or antianxiety medications are started, with very limited lasting effects. In an outpatient setting where the opportunity for observation of the patient is limited (as opposed to an inpatient unit where the patient can be observed 24 hours a day for several days by the staff), it is highly beneficial to get a history from significant others, especially in diagnosing disorders where externalization and denial are present. Thus, it is always beneficial to obtain information from the spouse or the parent of a patient. If a patient refuses to give permission to the clinician to obtain information from a supportive family member, the reason for the refusal should be explored fully. In general, such a refusal should be considered prima facie evidence of paranoia.

The anger, constricted affect, emotional sensitivity, and stubbornness seen in paranoid personalities partially respond to low doses of antidepressants, particularly the serotonergic antidepressants. The concurrent administration of an antidepressant helps keep the dose of an antipsychotic low; however, the antipsychotic is the primary medication in the treatment of paranoid personality disorder. An antidepressant is not necessary, but is usually beneficial.

Risperidone and olanzapine are the best choices as the first-line antipsychotic medications among currently available antipsychotics. Their favorable side effect profiles compared to traditional antipsychotics make them especially suitable for use in patients with personality disorders.

Case #2

Presenting Symptoms: The patient was a 50-year-old female, with symptoms of depressed mood, increased anxiety, irritability, moodiness, anxiety attacks, initial insomnia, frequent crying episodes, anergia, suicidal ideation, anhedonia, and feelings of hopelessness. The patient also had long-standing symptoms such as excessive emotional sensitivity, distrust of people, mild paranoid ideation and fears, introversion, scattered thinking, hypersensitivity to criticism, and a tendency to be suspicious of the motives of others. She denied drug and alcohol abuse. She reported smoking one-half pack of cigarettes per day and drinking six to eight cups of coffee daily. She was taking fluoxetine 20 mg AM for one year when she was first seen at my office. The patient had had two marriages. Her second divorce was 20 years ago, after which she chose to remain unmarried to avoid any close relationships. She denied any family history of psychiatric disorders. Her medical history is significant for fibromyalgia.

Axis II Diagnosis: Paranoid personality disorder

Axis I Diagnosis: Major depression, moderate, single episode

Current Treatment:
1. paroxetine 40 mg AM
2. risperidone 0.5 mg HS
3. zolpidem 2.5 mg HS PRN
4. psychotherapy
5. decrease coffee intake to two cups or less daily

Treatment Course: The dose of fluoxetine was increased to 40 mg AM at the first office visit. The patient was also started on risperidone 0.5 mg HS. Since the depressive symptoms did not improve when the patient was seen two weeks later, it was decided to discontinue fluoxetine and switch the patient to paroxetine 20 mg AM. Paroxetine was eventually increased to 40 mg AM for optimal resolution of depressive symptoms. Risperidone has been maintained at 0.5 mg HS. Both depressive and paranoid symptoms have shown satisfactory improvement. Zolpidem 2.5 mg is now used only as needed for occasional insomnia.

Comments: The patient's paranoid personality disorder was able to be diagnosed and treated because she presented for treatment of depression. In nearly all cases, patients' presenting complaints relate to Axis I symptoms. Personality disorder symptoms are not volunteered by the patient, but are elicited by the clinician from a longitudinal history. Collateral data from significant others are also helpful in understanding a patient's personality pattern because many of the dysfunctional aspects of a personality disorder are manifested in interpersonal relationships and in observable behavior.

This patient's paranoid personality could have predisposed her to depression. It must be extremely stressful for a patient to live with a chronic paranoid attitude that ultimately takes its toll emotionally, precipitating a depression or an anxiety disorder.

An analysis of this patient's symptoms revealed the presence of four symptom groups, which were addressed with medication as follows:

Symptom Group	Medication Class	Specific Medication
Depression	antidepressant	paroxetine 40 mg AM
Paranoid personality	antipsychotic	risperidone 0.5 mg HS
Anxiety, panic attacks	antidepressant (primary), anxiolytic (secondary)	paroxetine 40 mg AM
Insomnia	sedative-hypnotic	zolpidem 2.5 mg HS PRN

Both depression and anxiety can be effectively treated using antidepressants. Paroxetine improved both of these symptom groups in this patient. Appropriate treatment of Axis I and Axis II symptoms eventually improves peripheral symptoms such as insomnia and anorexia without specific treatment of these symptoms except during the first two to four weeks.

Case #3

Presenting Symptoms: The patient was a 33-year-old female, whose symptoms consisted of mood swings, depressed mood, occasional hypomanic episodes, paranoid ideation, episodic auditory hallucinations, suspiciousness, excessive emotional sensitivity, anger outbursts, distrust of others, perfectionistic tendencies, stubbornness, obsessive rumination, scattered thinking, and anxiety. These symptoms had been present since adolescence, with periodic exacerbations. The patient was pressured by her husband into coming for psychiatric treatment. She denied drug and alcohol abuse. She reported smoking one pack of cigarettes per day and drinking one to two cups of coffee daily. She had tried fluoxetine in the past but stopped after three days due to severe nausea. The patient's brother had been diagnosed with schizophrenia, and her grandmother suffered from depression. This patient's medical history was unremarkable.

Axis II Diagnosis:	Paranoid personality disorder with schizotypal and obsessive-compulsive personality features
Axis I Diagnosis:	Possible cyclothymia
Current Treatment:	1. trifluoperazine 2 mg HS 2. clomipramine 75 mg HS 3. carbamazepine 200 mg BID 4. psychotherapy

Treatment Course: The patient was treated with paroxetine, lorazepam, and risperidone, which were discontinued due to side effects. The combination of trifluoperazine (antipsychotic), clomipramine (antidepressant/antiobsessional), and carbamazepine (mood stabilizer) provided satisfactory resolution of all symptoms. Her carbamazepine level was 6 mcg/mL (6-12 mcg/mL).

Comments: Most personality disorders are treatable using combinations of medications that address the specific symptom clusters. In this case the medications treated the symptom groups listed:

Medication	Medication Class	Symptom Group
trifluoperazine	antipsychotic	paranoid, schizotypal
clomipramine	antidepressant	obsessive-compulsive personality symptoms, depression, anxiety
carbamazepine	mood stabilizer	mood instability, hypomanic episodes

It should be noted that both trifluoperazine and clomipramine are prescribed in low doses. For treatment of most personality disorders, low doses are desirable and sufficient.

Case #4

Presenting Symptoms: The patient was a 27-year-old female, with complaints of paranoia, racing thoughts, pressured speech, hostility when frustrated, reckless spending, labile affect, ideas of reference, and insomnia. She denied suicidal or homicidal ideation. The patient suffered marked deterioration in personal and occupational functioning over the last seven years, despite having a college degree. History from family members revealed that the patient had always been somewhat suspicious, secretive, emotionally sensitive, and distrustful. She had been noncompliant with taking antipsychotics and lithium, which were prescribed by other psychiatrists in the past. She denied drug and alcohol abuse, and caffeine intake. She reported smoking one pack of cigarettes per day. The patient's uncle had had several "nervous breakdowns."

Axis II Diagnosis: Paranoid personality disorder, premorbid (based on history obtained from a close family member)

Axis I Diagnosis: Schizoaffective disorder, bipolar type
Consider bipolar disorder
Consider schizophrenia, paranoid type
Consider delusional disorder, persecutory type

Current Treatment:
1. The patient refused voluntary hospitalization, which was recommended at the first visit.
2. Risperidone and lithium were prescribed as an outpatient treatment option, but the patient did not return after the first visit.

Treatment Course: The patient's family requested that she be hospitalized. Since she refused voluntary hospitalization and since she did not meet the clinical criteria for involuntary hospitalization at the time, she was offered outpatient treatment. The patient's family members, which included a physician, were upset that the author did not initiate involuntary commitment. The patient failed to keep her next appointment.

Comments: The major problem one encounters in treating patients with poor insight, including those with paranoid personality disorder, is their refusal to seek and/or accept treatment, and their noncompliance. With the recent availability of safer and more effective medications that have fewer side effects, some of the most difficult patients can be treated if treatment recommendations are followed by the patients. Most personality disorders (antisocial personality disorder is the notable exception) respond in varying degrees to a medication or combination of medications that are currently available. The problem is getting them to seek treatment and to comply with treatment recommendations.

Mental health professionals occasionally encounter cases like the one described above. The patient is chronically mentally ill and would benefit from inpatient treatment. This patient probably would have done well on clozapine, olanzapine, or risperidone, along with a mood stabilizer. The family's frustration and reaction are entirely justified and understandable, yet all patients, including the severely and chronically mentally ill, have the right to refuse treatment. All states provide for evaluating and treating a psychiatric patient involuntarily under strict conditions, which vary from state to state. However, most states allow involuntary commitment and treatment only if one of the following criteria is met:

1. The patient has threatened to harm him or herself, others, or property, due to mental illness.
2. The patient has attempted to or did harm him or herself, others, or property, due to mental illness.
3. The patient has been or will be imminently incapable of caring for him or herself, risking serious personal harm, due to mental illness.

Most states do not allow involuntary commitment even if extreme and overwhelming negative personal consequences have occurred or are imminent due to mental illness. Examples include giving away one's belongings and money in a manic state, or resigning from a stable job based on paranoid beliefs, or other extremely irrational acts.

In the absence of meeting such strict criteria, as required by individual states, the physician has no legal basis to commit a patient involuntarily—even if the physician feels that the patient needs inpatient treatment and the family demands it. The presence of severe mental illness alone is not sufficient for initiating involuntary commitment. Similarly, harming oneself or others is not sufficient to commit someone involuntarily to a psychiatric facility. For instance, a terminal patient expected to live for several months would not be psychiatrically hospitalized involuntarily in the absence of severe depression or psychosis, despite suicidal ideation or attempts. Also, people who assault others or commit murder are usually placed in jail rather than committed to a psychiatric hospital.

The clinician's duty is to apply clinical criteria and clinical judgment to individual cases to decide whether or not the patient meets the particular state's legal guidelines for involuntary commitment. Determination at a later time as to whether or not the patient met the legal criteria for involuntary commitment is the responsibility of the court system.

Although the physician's ultimate goal of making people well is noble, the means to achieving the goal must follow the state's legal guidelines, taking into consideration the patient's right to refuse psychiatric evaluation and/or treatment, even if such refusal, based on irrational beliefs and lack of insight, is not in the best interest of the patient.

It is quite probable that this patient will suffer further deterioration and possible serious adverse consequences in the future and hence is expected to meet clinical criteria for involuntary commitment at a later date.

Chapter 3

Schizoid Personality Disorder

The diagnostic criteria for Schizoid Personality Disorder according to *DSM-IV* are given below.

DSM-IV *CRITERIA AND SYMPTOM CORRELATES*

A. A pervasive pattern of detachment from social relationships and a restricted range of expression of emotions in interpersonal settings, beginning by early adulthood and present in a variety of contexts, as indicated by four (or more) of the following:

1. Neither desires nor enjoys close relationships, including being part of a family.
2. Almost always chooses solitary activities.
3. Has little, if any, interest in having sexual experiences with another person.
4. Takes pleasure in few, if any, activities.
5. Lacks close friends or confidants other than first-degree relatives.
6. Appears indifferent to the praise or criticism of others.
7. Shows emotional coldness, detachment, or flattened affectivity.

B. Does not occur exclusively during the course of schizophrenia, a mood disorder with psychotic features, another psychotic disorder, or a pervasive developmental disorder and is not due to the direct physiological effects of a general medical condition.

The approximate symptom correlates for each of the (overlapping) schizoid personality features are given in Table 3.1.

An analysis of the symptom correlates suggests that there are several symptoms that are potentially responsive to medication. Most of these symptoms resemble the "negative" or "deficit" symptoms of schizophrenia, consisting of emotional apathy, social withdrawal, blunted affect, constricted affect, anhedonia, dysphoria, poverty of speech and thought, avolition, and slowed thinking. Hence, theoretically, medications that improve the negative symptoms of schizophrenia should improve symptoms in schizoid personality disorder. The symptoms that need treatment and the medications that are thought to be effective are given here.

TABLE 3.1. Symptom Correlates for Schizoid Personality Disorder

DSM-IV **Criteria**	**Possible Symptom Correlates**
1. Neither desires nor enjoys close relationships, including being part of a family	social withdrawal, fear of intimacy, social anxiety, decreased social motivation, avoidant behavior
2. Almost always chooses solitary activities	seclusiveness
3. Has little, if any, interest in having sexual experiences with another person	decreased libido, dysphoria
4. Takes pleasure in few, if any, activities	anhedonia
5. Lacks close friends or confidants other than first-degree relatives	social inadequacy
6. Appears indifferent to the praise or criticism of others	blunted affect
7. Shows emotional coldness, detachment, or flattened affect	blunted affect

Symptom Cluster	Medications
Social withdrawal, blunted affect, seclusiveness, decreased social motivation, social inadequacy	low dose of risperidone, 0.5 to 1 mg QD olanzapine 2.5 to 5 mg HS
Anhedonia, decreased libido	nefazodone 200 to 500 mg QD bupropion 100 to 400 mg QD
Social anxiety	SSRIs and TCAs MAOIs low dose benzodiazepines beta-blockers

Clozapine, olanzapine, sertindole, and risperidone are the four antipsychotics that are most effective in improving deficit symptoms, and are likely to be of significant benefit to patients with schizoid personality disorder. However, given clozapine's risk of agranulocytosis, the use of clozapine would not be prudent unless the patient was significantly dysfunctional, in which case the diagnosis would most likely be schizophrenia or what was formerly known as simple schizophrenia. Even a low dose of clozapine puts the patient at risk for agranulocytosis. Therefore, for conditions that do not cause severe dysfunction, such as schizoid personality disorder, clozapine would not be a practical option, though I believe, from a theoretical standpoint, low doses of clozapine in combination with an antidepressant should significantly improve symptoms in this disorder. Concerning treatment effectiveness and symptom resolution alone, clozapine has the potential to be the most effective medication for the management of schizoid personality disorder. However, clozapine does not have FDA approval for treatment of schizoid personality disorder.

A practical solution is a trial of low doses of risperidone, olanzapine, or sertindole, which improves both positive and negative symptoms. Although risperidone's effectiveness for alleviating negative symptoms is not as strong as that of clozapine, in the author's experience it is clearly superior to traditional antipsychotics. The effectiveness of risperidone for positive symptoms seems to be greater than for negative symptoms. The recommended dose for optimal improvement in both positive and negative symptoms is 6 mg per day, which would be an excessive dose for patients with schizoid personality disorder, given the relative absence of positive symptoms in these individuals. For the above reasons, a low dose of risperidone at 0.5 to 1 mg per day is, by itself, not likely to give dramatic results in treating schizoid individuals. Olanzapine and sertindole, expected to be available in the future, might also be excellent choices. Once the neurochemical basis of negative symptoms is better understood, more specific treatment options will become available for use with people who have predominant negative symptoms (as with those suffering from schizoid personality disorder) and with people who have both positive and negative symptoms (those suffering from schizophrenia). Yet, physicians have an obligation to attempt to improve patients' quality of life and to decrease dysfunction through judicious and safe use of currently available treatment options. If risperidone, olanzapine, or sertindole at low doses are not effective or are not tolerated by the patient, other antipsychotics are not likely to be effective for treatment of schizoid personality disorder since other antipsychotics, with the exception of clozapine, are not particularly effective for the treatment of negative symptoms. Fortunately, antidepressants, particularly serotonergic antidepressants and bupropion, can improve negative symptoms to some extent. Perhaps negative symptoms represent a form of depression. In any case, schizoid individuals have symptoms of dysphoria, apathy, anhedonia, and decreased libido.

The decrease in libido in these patients is probably primary since it is believed that there is a paucity of sexual intimacy even if a mate is readily available, as in the case of a married couple. This suggests at least partial biological mediation, as for major depression. Hence, a trial of bupropion, which has energizing effects and which is relatively free of sexual side effects, has the potential to improve depressive symptoms and sexual functioning in schizoid individuals.

Social anxiety can be treated by using serotonergic antidepressants although historically MAOIs have been effectively used for this condition. (With the anticipated introduction of second generation, highly selective MAOIs such as moclobemide and braforamine, some of the dietary restrictions and medication interaction risks are not expected to be of concern.) A low dose of alprazolam at 0.25 to 0.5 mg TID, or adjunctive use of beta blockers such as propranolol LA 60 to 120 mg per day or atenolol 50 to 100 mg per day are other medication options which may be used in combination with an antidepressant and an antipsychotic to reduce social anxiety.

People with schizoid personality disorder come to the physician at the urging of concerned close family members. They require continued persuasion from the family members and active encouragement from the physician to stay in treatment, especially in the initial stages of medication trials. Once their social discomfort has improved with treatment and they realize the benefits, they are likely to be more motivated to stay in treatment. The treatment is expected to be fairly long-term.

Social-skills training is a form of cognitive-behavioral therapy that is helpful to people who are socially inadequate or those who experience social anxiety, as in the case of schizoid personality disorder. Individual psychotherapy is also helpful as long as the therapist is fairly directive and active in a supportive and concrete therapeutic framework. However, in order to maximally benefit from social-skills training and psychotherapy, the schizoid patient should ideally first be treated on a balanced combination of medications as suggested earlier in this chapter. Dosage ranges of various medication combinations for healthy adults are given here.

- risperidone 0.5 to 1 mg QD
- olanzapine 2.5 to 5 mg HS
- fluoxetine 20 to 40 mg (or any of the serotonergic antidepressants, MAOIs, or bupropion)
- alprazolam 0.25 mg TID or QID
- propranolol LA 60 mg QAM

Risperidone and olanzapine have the potential to improve negative symptoms. Antidepressants should treat anhedonia, social anxiety, anergia, and overall dysphoria. Social anxiety, in addition, might respond to alprazolam, or to beta blockers such as propranolol or atenolol. Since psychiatric problems are composed of unique clusters of symptoms, each of which responds to different medications, it is necessary to use combinations of medications to address the various distinct symptom clusters.

Physicians should be familiar with understanding patients' problems in terms of component symptoms for selection of effective treatments, whereas an interpersonal, behavioral, or psychodynamic understanding will help a psychotherapist to select different psychotherapeutic approaches and techniques that are appropriate for a particular patient. Psychological understanding of the patient will help the physician deal with patients, and anticipate their resistances and defenses thereby ensuring compliance with, and success of, medication treatment. It is, therefore, important for a physician prescribing psychiatric medications to understand the psychology of the individual patient in order to facilitate medication treatment. It is the author's observation that even biologically oriented psychiatrists are more effective and are better accepted by patients if they are able to understand the patients' psychodynamic and interpersonal issues. The expectation is that understanding of the patients' psychological dynamics will enable the physician to anticipate and manage medication resistance and noncompliance before they undermine treatment. Various practical aspects of the diagnosis and treatment of schizoid personality disorder are illustrated in Cases 5, 6, 7, and 8.

A complete resolution of schizoid symptoms is not a realistic goal. Even with effective treatment, schizoid patients remain introverted. The treatment goal should be to decrease the severity of the dysfunctional symptoms.

CLINICAL CASES 5 to 8

Case #5

Presenting Symptoms: The patient was a 28-year-old male whose symptoms consisted of seclusiveness, extreme social withdrawal and shyness, excessive preference for solitary activities, avoidance of intimacy, flat affect, anergia, apathy, and anhedonia. These symptoms emerged during late adolescence. Treatment was initiated after considerable pressure from family members, who took the initiative to bring him for treatment and to ensure that he was taking the medications. He denied drug and alcohol abuse, and smoking. He reported drinking two cups of coffee daily. His father had a seizure disorder and possible schizophrenia, simple type. His sister was described as "very shy." The patient quit working about a year prior to starting treatment because he did not like interacting with people. He denied any history of major medical problems.

Axis II Diagnosis: Schizoid personality disorder

Current Treatment: 1. risperidone 1 mg AM and 2 mg HS
2. fluoxetine 20 mg AM
3. psychotherapy (not fully compliant)

Treatment Course: The patient was started on risperidone 0.5 mg BID at the first visit and the dose was gradually increased over a period of one month to 1 mg AM and 2 mg HS. Seclusiveness, social withdrawal, flat affect, and shyness improved, but apathy and anhedonia persisted; therefore, fluoxetine was added after about two months of treatment. Further improvement in all of the schizoid symptoms were noted two weeks after starting fluoxetine. The patient improved and was able to return to work. He is still introverted, but not as dysfunctional.

Comments: Diagnostically, this patient could be classified as suffering from simple schizophrenia, which currently is not a formal *DSM-IV* diagnosis. The criteria set for simple schizophrenia (formally called simple deteriorative disorder) is described in *DSM-IV* in Appendix B, titled "Criteria Sets and Axes Provided for Further Study," and is summarized below.

Criteria for simple deteriorative disorder (simple schizophrenia): Gradual onset and progressive deterioration of all of the following symptoms over a one-year period:

1. Marked decline in occupational or academic functioning
2. Negative symptoms such as flat affect, alogia, and avolition
3. Poor interpersonal rapport, social isolation, or social withdrawal

The criteria set for simple deteriorative disorder also requires that the patient should not have any of the characteristic symptoms of schizophrenia such as delusions, hallucinations, disorganized speech, and grossly disorganized or catatonic behavior. It is unlikely that, without the active interest and initiative by the family members, this patient would have accepted treatment. Resistance to treatment is unfortunately true of nearly all personality disorders, as is also generally true with some of the Axis I disorders such as schizophrenia, manic phase of bipolar disorder, delusional disorders, paraphilias, and substance abuse.

If the dysfunction and the negative symptoms are severe, use of clozapine may be considered because, in the author's opinion, clozapine has better effectiveness for treating negative symptoms compared to all other antipsychotics currently available. Risperidone's effect on negative symptoms is superior to that of traditional antipsychotics. Therefore, risperidone serves as an excellent first-line general purpose antipsychotic, besides olanzapine.

SSRIs tend to improve social anxiety, social phobia, social introversion, apathy, anhedonia, and affective flattening which, in addition to being schizoid characteristics, might represent a mild form of negative symptoms. The addition of a stimulating SSRI such as fluoxetine, sertraline, or venlafaxine might benefit patients with schizoid personality disorder or prominent negative symptoms. In individual cases, other SSRIs, TCAs, MAOIs, nefazodone, or bupropion might be effective.

Case #6

Presenting Symptoms: The patient was a 51-year-old male, whose symptoms consisted of depressed mood, anxiety, restless sleep, anergia, and a habit of drinking a fifth of vodka daily. Personality characteristics consisted of dislike of social interaction, anhedonia, social withdrawal, constricted affect, perfectionistic tendencies, excessive devotion to work, and stubbornness. No precipitants were identified by the patient. He denied drug abuse, smoking, and caffeine intake. His father suffered from "anxiety." The medical history is significant for borderline hypertension.

Axis II Diagnosis:	Schizoid personality disorder with obsessive-compulsive personality features
Axis I Diagnosis:	Dysthymia Alcohol dependence
Current Treatment:	1. paroxetine 30 mg AM 2. risperidone 0.5 mg HS 3. trazodone 50 mg HS 4. psychotherapy 5. referral to AA

Treatment Course: Tapering doses of chlordiazepoxide were given on an outpatient basis for the first five days to safely stop alcohol consumption. Concurrent treatment using paroxetine 10 mg AM and trazodone 50 mg HS was started on the day of the first visit to my office. The patient had no difficulty in withdrawing from alcohol with the help of chlordiazepoxide. The dose of paroxetine was increased to 20 mg AM at the next office visit ten days later. He reported moderate improvement but still complained of depressive and obsessional symptoms during his third office visit; thus, paroxetine was again increased to 30 mg with satisfactory improvement in obsessive-compulsive and depressive symptoms, and mild improvement in schizoid symptoms. When risperidone 0.5 mg HS was added, the schizoid symptoms further improved. This improvement has been sustained over several months. Naltrexone was offered to treat the patient's alcoholism but he felt that he could abstain without having to take naltrexone.

Comments: Discrete symptom groups and corresponding medications that benefitted this patient are given below.

Symptom Group	Medication Class	Specific Medication
Alcohol dependence	sedative	chlordiazepoxide (5 days) (naltrexone offered, but refused)
Schizoid symptoms	antipsychotic (antidepressant)*	risperidone 0.5 mg HS (paroxetine 30 mg HS)
Obsessive-compulsive personality traits	antiobsessional	paroxetine 30 mg AM
Insomnia	sedative-hypnotic	trazodone 50 mg HS

Trazodone is an antidepressant, not a sedative-hypnotic; however, since trazodone is employed in this case for its hypnotic properties, it is classified as a sedative-hypnotic in a functional sense. The patient's dislike of social interaction, constricted affect, and social withdrawal have become less intense with this treatment.

Case #7

Presenting Symptoms: The patient was a 32-year-old male, with complaints of irresistible exhibitionistic and voyeuristic urges, ob-

*Antidepressants are used as secondary medications in the treatment of schizoid personality disorder.

sessive preoccupation with pedophilia, conviction for child sexual molestation resulting in a ten-year probation, compulsive organizing, perfectionistic tendencies, schizoid tendencies, ideas of reference, extreme social withdrawal, depressed mood, and feelings of hopelessness. Extreme social introversion, obsessional characteristics, and pedophilic preoccupation have been present since adolescence. The patient presented for the psychiatric evaluation because he was required to do so by a probation stipulation. He denied drug and alcohol abuse, smoking, and caffeine intake. He also denied a family history of psychiatric disorders. The patient had never been married.

Axis II Diagnosis: Schizoid personality disorder with obsessive-compulsive, schizotypals and antisocial features

Axis I Diagnosis: Pedophilia
Obsessive-Compulsive disorder

Current Treatment:
1. paroxetine 45 mg HS
2. risperidone 1 mg HS
3. continue counseling (required by probation department)

Treatment Course: At the first visit the patient was started on paroxetine 20 mg AM and risperidone 0.5 mg HS. Remarkable improvement was reported by the patient at the second office visit two weeks later. Paroxetine was increased to 30 mg HS and risperidone increased to 1 mg HS at the second visit for an even more effective response. Paroxetine was further increased to 45 mg to control residual obsessive preoccupation with pedophilia. According to the patient's report, there was a dramatic improvement in all of his symptoms. Paroxetine was switched to bedtime dosage to capitalize on the sedation experienced by the patient during the daytime.

Comments: This patient's symptoms point to a multitude of diagnostic possibilities. On the Axis I level, the patient clearly has pedophilia, and probably obsessive-compulsive disorder. The patient also has a personality disorder that the author suspects is predominantly characterized by schizoid features with obsessive-compulsive, schizotypal, and antisocial tendencies. Another psychiatrist could reasonably diagnose other mixtures of personality characteristics; however, accurate identification of important symptoms is sufficient for practical treatment to begin.

Patients who are already convicted of a crime and who seek psychiatric treatment as required by the court system are usually not genuinely motivated. They tend to minimize their psychiatric history and be superficially cooperative to fulfill the requirements imposed by the court. On the other hand, patients who seek psychiatric evaluation and treatment in the course of litigation generally exaggerate psychiatric pathology, if any secondary legal gains are possible. All things considered, the patients who seek psychiatric treatment after a conviction or after legal issues are settled tend to benefit more from psychiatric intervention because of absence of major secondary gains. In view of these general observations, it is possible that this patient is exaggerating the extent of improvement so that he can fulfill his legal obligations. However, his facial expression, eye contact, voice characteristics, physical manner and appearance, and feedback from his counselor (who has known him for many months) suggest that the medication intervention has had genuine positive effects.

The patient claimed that his social withdrawal, social anxiety, fears, obsessional tendencies, pedophilic preoccupation, and paranoia, which he admitted had been present since early adolescence, had nearly completely faded. The author believes that the medication significantly suppressed his Axis I and Axis II symptoms. The symptom analysis and medication choice are summarized below.

Symptom Group	Medication Group	Specific Medication
Pedophilia, obsessive-compulsive symptoms, exhibitionism, voyeurism	antiobsessional (SSRIs, clomipramine)	paroxetine
Schizoid, schizotypal, paranoid symptoms	antipsychotic	risperidone
Depression	antidepressant	paroxetine

The varied symptoms belonging to Axes I and II are reduced to compatible groupings of symptoms and treated using specific medications to address the symptom groups. The clinical process of reducing a variety of symptoms to a small group of treatable symptom groups is more fundamentally important than the specific choice of medications. For instance, another psychiatrist could have chosen clomipramine and thiothixene and perhaps have had a similar, better, or worse result. However, failure to identify the fundamental symptom clusters will most likely result in a suboptimal treatment outcome.

Case #8

Presenting Symptoms: The patient was a 21-year-old male, with symptoms consisting of social withdrawal, seclusiveness, dislike of social interaction, anhedonia, anergia, depressed mood, apathy, difficulty focusing thoughts, poor concentration, distractibility, and excessive worrying. He denied drug and alcohol abuse, and caffeine intake. He reported smoking one-half pack of cigarettes per day. The patient was prescribed thioridazine for a brief period at age 13 for unknown reasons. He denied major medical problems. The above symptoms at less severity have been present since early adolescence.

Axis II Diagnosis: Schizoid personality disorder

Axis I Diagnosis: Attention deficit disorder (ADD)
Dysthymia

Current Treatment:
1. bupropion 100 mg TID
2. fluoxetine 20 mg AM
3. risperidone 0.5 mg HS
4. referral for psychotherapy

Treatment Course: Bupropion was started at 100 mg AM and gradually increased to 100 mg BID, leading to improvement in ADD symptoms and dysthymia. Addition of risperidone 0.5 mg HS and fluoxetine 20 mg AM resulted in improvement in schizoid symptoms.

Comments: For schizoid symptoms, a combination of a low dose of an antipsychotic and a medium dose of an antidepressant are somewhat effective. Schizoid individuals are not expected to become extroverted, but symptoms such as social withdrawal, apathy, seclusiveness and anhedonia may show moderate improvement.

There is a depressive component to typical symptoms associated with schizoid personality disorder. These symptoms tend to overlap with that of dysthymia and the negative symptoms of schizophrenia. Atypical antipsychotics such as risperidone, olanzapine, and clozapine should be particularly effective, along with antidepressant medication (preferably SSRIs) for treatment of disorders having predominantly negative symptoms.

Chapter 4

Schizotypal Personality Disorder

DSM-IV criteria for diagnosis of schizotypal personality disorder are given below.

DSM-IV *CRITERIA AND SYMPTOM CORRELATES*

A. A pervasive pattern of social and interpersonal deficits marked by acute discomfort with, and reduced capacity for, close relationships as well as by cognitive or perceptual distortions and eccentricities of behavior, beginning in early adulthood and present in a variety of contexts, as indicated by five (or more) of the following:

1. *Ideas of reference (excluding delusions of reference).*
2. *Odd beliefs or magical thinking that influences behavior and is inconsistent with subcultural norms (e.g., superstitiousness, belief in clairvoyance, telepathy, or "sixth sense"; in children and adolescents, bizarre fantasies or preoccupations).*
3. *Unusual perceptual experiences, including bodily illusions.*
4. *Odd thinking and speech (e.g., vague, circumstantial, metaphorical, overelaborate, or stereotyped).*
5. *Suspiciousness or paranoid ideation.*
6. *Inappropriate or constricted affect.*
7. *Behavior or appearance that is odd, eccentric, or peculiar.*
8. *Lack of close friends or confidants other than first-degree relatives.*

---

9. Excessive social anxiety that does not diminish with familiarity and tends to be associated with paranoid fears rather than negative judgments about self.

B. Does not occur exclusively during the course of schizophrenia, a mood disorder with psychotic features, another psychotic disorder, or a pervasive developmental disorder.

The symptom correlates corresponding to *DSM-IV* criteria are noted in Table 4.1.

An analysis of the symptom correlates suggests two major symptom clusters and one minor symptom cluster that could respond to two different classes of medications.

Symptom Cluster	Medication
Ideas of reference, disorder of thinking, perceptual disorder, paranoia	antipsychotics (primary)
Obsessional and compulsive features, social anxiety	serotonergic antidepressants, clomipramine, MAOIs
Deficit symptoms–social withdrawal, constricted affect	SSRIs, atypical antipsychotics

Comparative analysis from a symptom standpoint reveals that among paranoid, schizoid and schizotypal personality disorders (Cluster A), paranoid personality disorder typically has fairly equal psychotic and obsessional symptom intensity, schizoid disorders have predominantly depressive symptoms consisting of negative or deficit symptoms with significant social anxiety, and schizotypal disorders have primarily psychotic symptoms and a mild degree of obsessive-compulsive and deficit features. Strictly from a symptomatic approach, schizotypal personality disorder can be considered a mild form of schizophrenia with the same characteristics except that psychotic thought, perceptual, and affective symptoms are mild; hence the personal, social, and occupational deterioration

TABLE 4.1. Symptom Correlates for Schizotypal Personality Disorder

	***DSM-IV* Criteria**	**Possible Symptom Correlates**
1.	Ideas of reference (excluding delusions of reference)	ideas of reference (psychotic symptom)
2.	Odd beliefs or magical thinking that influences behavior and is inconsistent with subcultural norms (e.g., superstitiousness, belief in clairvoyance, telepathy, or "sixth sense"; in children and adolescents, bizarre fantasies or preoccupations)	obsessional and compulsive features
3.	Unusual perceptual experiences, including bodily illusions	perceptual distortion (psychotic symptom)
4.	Odd thinking and speech (e.g., vague, circumstantial, metaphorical, overelaborate, or stereotyped)	thought disorder (psychotic symptom)
5.	Suspiciousness and paranoid ideation	paranoia (psychotic symptom)
6.	Inappropriate or constricted affect	deficit symptoms (depressive tendency)
7.	Behavior or appearance that is odd, eccentric, or peculiar	thought disorder (psychotic symptom)
8.	Lack of close friends or confidants other than first-degree relatives	social withdrawal (depressive tendency)
9.	Excessive social anxiety that does not diminish with familiarity and tends to be associated with paranoid fears rather than negative judgments about self	social anxiety

are proportionately less severe. The notion that schizotypal symptoms and more severe psychosis are in a continuum is illustrated in Figure 4.1. Since the difference is quantitative and not qualitative, the treatment employs similar medications, the primary difference being in the dose size. It is a general clinical observation that, as

FIGURE 4.1. Normalcy-Psychosis Continuum

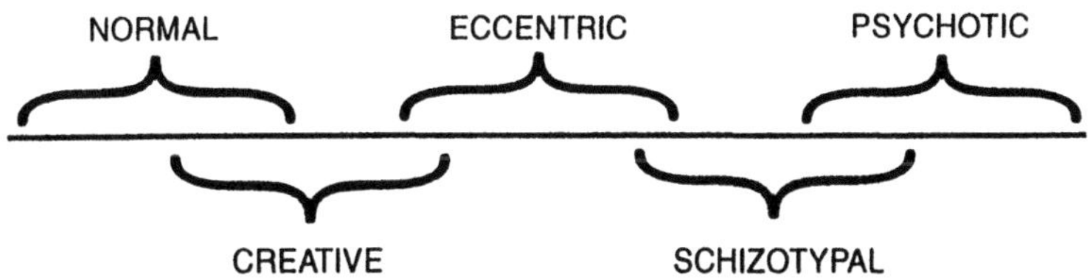

noted earlier, the therapeutic effects of medication and the extent of side effects are in a continuum, with a greater degree of efficacy and greater side effects as the dosage is increased, with some poorly understood exceptions as in the case of nortriptyline, and to some extent for risperidone, for which there is thought to be a range of optimal blood level and dosage.

The schizotypal personality disorder can be more effectively treated than can schizophrenia, using medications such as clozapine, risperidone, olanzapine, and sertindole for both positive and negative symptoms. Since the symptoms of schizotypal personality disorder are not as florid as those of schizophrenia and since the symptoms do not cause severe dysfunction, clozapine is not typically used for treatment of schizotypal personality disorder. However, from a fundamental neuropharmacological standpoint, clozapine at low doses should be a superior medication for treating schizotypal symptoms. It is the author's observation that most schizophrenics have at various times manifestations of obsessive and compulsive features, as well as depressive features. The depressive symptoms can be manifestations of negative symptoms, demoralization secondary to having a chronic illness, or side effects of medications (e.g., akinesia). Serotonergic antidepressants can improve both obsessive and compulsive symptoms and depressive symptoms that are commonly found in patients with schizotypal personality disorder and schizophrenia. It is emphasized again that antidepressants in the absence of antipsychotics can make the psychosis worse in patients who have underlying psychosis. Examples of various combination treatment for schizotypal personality disorder are given below.

1. risperidone 1 mg HS
   clomipramine 50-100 mg HS
2. olanzapine 5 mg HS
   fluvoxamine 100 mg HS
3. haloperidol 2 mg HS
   nefazodone 100 mg TID
4. any of the antipsychotics at low doses
   any of the antidepressants (SSRIs preferred due to their benign side effect profile)

As with any other patient, the adjunctive need for anticholinergic medication, hypnotics, or appetite stimulants may arise in which case these additional medications are added as needed. The recommended first-line antipsychotic are risperidone, olanzapine, and sertindole because of the low risk of extrapyramidal symptoms (EPS) and other neuroleptic side effects. There is an expectation that risperidone, olanzapine, and sertindole, in addition to having less acute side effects, have less risk of causing tardive dyskinesia compared to traditional antipsychotics. Whether or not this expectation will materialize will be known only with years of experience. As discussed above, medication effectiveness is not an all-or-none phenomenon. In everyday clinical practice, it is a common observation that mild problems respond satisfactorily to low doses, and severe symptoms respond to dosages at the higher end of the dosage range. In real life there is no absolute dose that is subtherapeutic for everybody. Dosage must be individualized. What is subtherapeutic for one patient can be the optimal or even toxic dose for another patient.

Since the severity of psychotic, obsessive-compulsive, and depressive symptoms are mild in schizotypal personality disorder compared to schizophrenia, lower doses of the antipsychotics and antidepressants should be effective. Schizotypal patients can present with complaints of depression and anxiety; thus, it is important to obtain a thorough history and mental status examination and–perhaps more importantly–obtain collateral information to discover other underlying problems. Several clinical cases of schizotypal personality disorder are presented and discussed in this text. These cases illustrate the practical application of clinical concepts and pharmacological techniques outlined above.

CLINICAL CASES 9 to 16

Case #9

Presenting Symptoms: The patient was a 50-year-old female, whose symptoms consisted of scattered thinking, poor concentration, poor memory, intermittent yelling while asleep, occasional auditory hallucinations, paranoia, ideas of reference, obsessive ruminations, mild compulsive organizing and cleaning, concrete thinking, rigid beliefs, depressed mood, and insomnia. These symptoms had been present since early adulthood. She denied drug and alcohol abuse, smoking, and caffeine intake. The patient also denied any previous psychiatric evaluation or treatment. Her brother and mother suffered from "chronic mental illness." The medical history is significant for mitral valve prolapse, asthma, and peripheral vascular disease. This patient was taking dipyridamole 50 mg TID, propranolol 10 mg BID, and theophylline 100 mg BID.

Axis II Diagnosis: Schizotypal personality disorder with obsessive-compulsive features

Current Treatment:
1. fluoxetine 40 mg AM
2. risperidone 1 mg BID
3. temazepam 15 mg HS
4. psychotherapy

Treatment Course: At the first visit, the patient was started on risperidone 0.5 mg HS, fluoxetine 10 mg AM, and temazepam 15 mg HS. She reported mild improvement at the second visit, three weeks later. The dose of fluoxetine was gradually increased to the current dose of 40 mg. Risperidone was ultimately increased to 1 mg BID, over a period of ten weeks. The patient reported almost complete resolution of most symptoms and felt that she should have started this treatment 25 years ago.

Comments: The new generation antidepressants (SSRIs, venlafaxine, clomipramine, nefazodone, and bupropion) and antipsychotics (risperidone, olanzapine, and clozapine) were not available 25 years ago so the patient could not have been started on these medications. A number of tricyclic antidepressants (TCAs), MAOIs and traditional antipsychotics were available 20 to 25 years ago but had the disadvantage of an unfavorable side effect profile, which interfered with medication compliance.

With most personality disorder patients it is particularly important to start at very low doses for several reasons:

- Their symptoms are usually not severe.
- They typically seek help due to external pressures; thus, even a mild side effect can serve as an excuse to devalue and refuse medications. Minimization of side effects and acceptance of treatment are more important during the initial stages of treatment than is symptom resolution.
- Some patients (paranoid, narcissistic, for example) are very sensitive to side effects.

This patient was started on fluoxetine 10 mg and risperidone 0.5 mg HS, which are very low doses for both of these medications. She was kept on them for three weeks prior to any further increase. This clinical strategy may be contrasted with the treatment of an Axis I disorder such as psychosis, bipolar disorder, or depressive disorder where higher doses are typically employed as starting doses.

Symptom analysis revealed four discrete symptom groups as follows:

Symptom Group	Medication Group	Specific Medication
Schizotypal	antipsychotic	risperidone
Obsessive-compulsive	SSRIs	fluoxetine
Depressive	antidepressant	fluoxetine
Insomnia	hypnotic	temazepam

Any one of the many antipsychotics, antidepressants, and hypnotics could have been chosen and could have given equal (or even better) results. The important idea is to reduce the patient's presenting symptoms to one or more distinct symptom clusters and to choose a medication from one or more classes of psychotropics to treat all of the symptom groups. The choice of a specific medication within a class of medication is not as crucial in most cases. For example, instead of fluoxetine, another clinician could have chosen sertraline, paroxetine, venlafaxine, fluvoxamine or clomipramine, all of which are excellent for treatment of obsessive-compulsive symptoms and depression. Similarly, zolpidem, lorazepam, alprazolam, clonazepam, or trazodone would have been acceptable choices instead of temazepam. Risperidone and olanzapine, due to their improved side effect profile, currently have no competition for treatment of relatively mild psychotic symptoms (as in some personality disorders), and so are preferred as general purpose first-line antipsychotics.

Case #10

Presenting Symptoms: The patient was a 31-year-old male, whose symptoms consisted of grandiosity, circumstantial thinking, mood swings, obsessive-compulsive symptoms, hypomanic episodes, paranoia, overinclusive thinking, a history of several recent psychotic episodes, excessive preoccupation with order, stubbornness, and perfectionistic tendencies. Many of the symptoms at low severity had been present since his early teens. He had a history of episodic binge drinking. He denied drug abuse, smoking, or caffeine intake. The patient had been seen by at least six psychiatrists previously. Two of them felt that he primarily had a personality disorder. A compilation of previous diagnoses by various psychiatrists are as follows:

Axis I: Bipolar disorder
Cyclothymia
Schizophrenia
Schizoaffective disorder
Obsessive-compulsive disorder
Adjustment disorder with depressed mood

Axis II: Obsessive-compulsive personality disorder
Paranoid personality disorder
Personality disorder, not otherwise specified

He was treated with all classes of psychotropic medications, including lithium and haloperidol. There is a strong family history of psychiatric disorders. Both of his parents are believed to have had obsessive-compulsive personality disorder, if not obsessive-compulsive disorder. His brother had been diagnosed with paranoid schizophrenia. His grandmother was described as paranoid. The patient's medical history was unremarkable.

Axis II Diagnosis: Schizotypal personality disorder with obsessive-compulsive and paranoid features

Axis I Diagnosis: Schizoaffective disorder, bipolar type obsessive-compulsive disorder

Current Treatment:
1. paroxetine 45 mg AM
2. lithium carbonate 300 mg TID
3. risperidone 1.5 mg AM and 3 mg HS
4. lorazepam 0.5 mg BID PRN
5. benztropine 1 mg BID PRN
6. propranolol 10 mg TID PRN
7. psychotherapy

Treatment Course: The patient had stopped taking thiothixene 10 mg HS against medical advice. After about three months of stopping thiothixene, he had a severe manic/psychotic decompensation for which he was hospitalized and discharged after about ten days. He has been fairly stable on the current combination of medications. The personality disorder symptoms have shown moderate improvement so far. The option of switching to clozapine was discussed with the patient and his family. Because of financial difficulties, he is unable to pursue clozapine treatment at the present time. The author expects clozapine to give better results for this patient.

Comments: It is not unusual to find low diagnostic correlation among different clinicians when dealing with a complicated patient. Among Axis II diagnoses, any of the following diagnoses are reasonable for this patient:

Personality disorder, not otherwise specified (NOS)
Paranoid personality disorder with schizotypal and obsessive-compulsive features
Obsessive-compulsive personality disorder with schizotypal and paranoid features

The patient has symptoms which overlap *among* Axis I and Axis II disorders and *between* Axis I and Axis II disorders, making it difficult to arrive at a precise diagnosis that will be accepted unanimously by a group of psychiatrists. It is especially important to rely on specific symptoms rather than on diagnoses when treating a very complicated patient such as this patient, whereas for a straightforward diagnosis such as panic disorder with agoraphobia or obsessive-compulsive personality disorder, specific symptom analysis is perhaps not as crucial for purposes of psychopharmacological intervention.

Case #11

Presenting Symptoms: The patient was a 72-year-old female, with complaints of anxiety, depressed mood, episodic auditory hallucinations with persecutory content, insomnia, obsessive rumination, irritability, obsessive fear of dying, ideas of reference, and anhedonia. The patient revealed that she had been hearing voices since her late teens and avoided being home alone because of this. She stated that the voices had started again about four months prior to this office visit. Depressive symptoms emerged four months ago for the first time. The patient had been under stress due to her husband's cancer, which was discovered one year ago and which worsened six months ago. She denied drug and alcohol abuse, smoking, and caffeine intake. She also denied any previous psychiatric evaluation or treatment. This patient had hypertension and arthritis. She was taking metoprolol.

Axis II Diagnosis:	Schizotypal personality disorder with dependent features
Axis I Diagnosis:	Adjustment disorder with depressed mood and anxiety Consider psychosis, not otherwise specified (NOS)
Current Treatment:	1. risperidone 0.5 mg HS 2. clomipramine 25 mg HS 3. referral for psychotherapy

Treatment Course: Both clomipramine 25 mg HS and risperidone 0.5 mg HS were started at the first visit. When seen two weeks later, the patient reported remarkable improvement in all of the symptoms. Sustained improvement was seen two months later, with no side effects. She is now seen once every three months for medication management.

Comments: I am yet uncertain regarding this patient's Axis I diagnosis. Among Axis II diagnoses, she seems to meet the criteria for schizotypal personality disorder. She could be categorized as having schizophrenia, residual type; psychosis, NOS; or schizo-affective disorder, depressed. The symptoms–until recently–were of low severity, suggesting that she probably has a schizotypal personality disorder, temporarily worsened by the stress of her husband's terminal illness.

Because of her age, very low doses were initially prescribed. Fortunately, this worked well. The patient's symptoms improved to the point at which she is fully satisfied with the treatment. Since she is currently asymptomatic, there is no reason to increase the dose. Clomipramine was chosen to address the obsessional quality associated with her fear, anxiety, and depressed mood.

Case #12

Presenting Symptoms: The patient was a 63-year-old female, with complaints of increased anxiety, middle and terminal insomnia, distrust, dysphoria, excessive emotional sensitivity, superstitious beliefs, concrete religious preoccupation, suspiciousness, excessive praying, rigid beliefs, frequent audible conversation with herself, and emotional apathy. Increased anxiety and insomnia were the chief complaints. Additional information was obtained from a family member. Most of the symptoms have been present since early adulthood. She denied drug and alcohol abuse, smoking, and caffeine intake. She denied any acute precipitants. She also denied any previous psychiatric evaluation or treatment. The patient's sister had been diagnosed with schizophrenia. The patient had never been married. Her medical history is positive for Type II diabetes, for which she was taking glipizide 10 mg BID.

Axis II Diagnosis: Schizotypal personality disorder, with obsessional features

Current Treatment: 1. risperidone 0.25 mg (1/4th of a 1 mg pill) HS
2. fluoxetine 10 mg AM
3. zolpidem 5 mg HS PRN insomnia

Treatment Course: The patient was given risperidone 0.25 mg HS and fluoxetine 10 mg AM at the first visit. She was instructed to take zolpidem 5 mg if she woke up and was unable to resume sleep. Zolpidem was used only on the first several nights after which sleep normalized. Significant improvement in all of the symptoms with no side effects were reported at the second office visit two weeks later, so medication dosage was not changed.

Comments: This patient's symptoms fall under three discrete classes:

1. Mild psychotic symptoms
2. Mild obsessive-compulsive symptoms
3. Mild dysphoria

Anxiety and insomnia, which were the chief complaints, are probably secondary symptoms. The patient's excellent response to extremely low doses of an antipsychotic and an antiobsessional/antidepressant medication is instructive. Patients with personality disorders rarely present with the core symptoms of the personality disorder as the chief complaint. Rather, they present with chief complaints that are truly secondary and nonspecific, such as anxiety, dysphoria, insomnia, anorexia, anergia, apathy, anhedonia, anxiety attacks, etc. If the chief complaints of anxiety and insomnia are taken at face value, and if the treatment is aimed at directly alleviating these symptoms, the treatment is likely to consist of a benzodiazepine which, at best, is expected to be only partially or temporarily effective. Historical information from a significant other is crucial in obtaining the longitudinal perspective and the observational data necessary to diagnose a personality disorder. For example, antisocial, paranoid, and narcissistic patients are likely to be guarded and hence are unlikely to reveal detailed information necessary for the diagnosis. Obviously, without accurate identification of primary and secondary symptoms (leading to the correct diagnosis), appropriate treatment cannot be instituted.

This case illustrates the successful use of very small doses of medications for treating relatively mild symptoms. Most personality disorder symptoms can be successfully treated if patients are compliant, despite the fact that for the most part patients are initially brought to psychiatric attention due to persuasion by family members, employers, school, or the court system.

Case #13

Presenting Symptoms: The patient was a 28-year-old female, with complaints of difficulty organizing and focusing thoughts, vague thinking, feelings of having "close contacts" with people, avoidance of social situations, apathy, introversion, obsessive worrying, and seclusiveness. These symptoms have been present since her early teens. She was brought to the office by her parents with whom she lives. She works part-time as a sales clerk. She denied drug and alcohol abuse, smoking, and caffeine intake. She also denied a history of major medical problems.

Axis II Diagnosis: Schizotypal personality disorder with schizoid, obsessive, and dependent features

Current Treatment: 1. risperidone 1 mg HS
2. fluoxetine 20 mg AM

Treatment Course: The patient was initially started on risperidone 0.5 mg HS, and increased to her current dose of 1 mg HS, which improved thought disorganization and eccentric thinking. Fluoxetine was later added, starting at 10 mg and eventually increased to 20 mg, which significantly improved apathy, obsessive rumination, social withdrawal, and affective blunting.

Comments: Since treatment is predicated on symptoms, the treatment would be the same regardless of diagnosis. For example, this patient could conceivably be diagnosed as any one of the following:

Schizotypal personality disorder with schizoid, obsessive, and dependent features
Schizoid personality disorder with schizotypal, obsessional, and dependent features

Dependent personality disorder with schizotypal, schizoid, and obsessional features
Simple schizophrenia (proposed)

Another clinician could diagnose this patient with any of the above diagnoses, and possibly even schizophrenia, yet the patient is likely to need a combination of an antipsychotic and an antidepressant medication for optimal improvement. Personality disorders characterize lifelong patterns whereas most Axis I disorders require distinct deterioration from a higher level of premorbid or baseline functioning. This distinction is frequently difficult to make when dealing with mild forms of Axis I psychotic disorders and Cluster A personality disorders such as paranoid, schizotypal, and schizoid personality disorders. In most clinical contexts the symptoms of Axis I psychotic disorders and Cluster A personality disorders do not manifest until patients reach their teens. For the most part this differentiation has no significant practical impact because if symptoms are mild, treatment is usually the same. If psychotic symptoms are prominent, the diagnosis is generally in the Axis I level, and the treatment could call for clozapine as a primary medication. Generally, a low dose of medication is sufficient for treating personality disorders, the exception being borderline personality disorder.

Case #14

Presenting Symptoms: The patient was a 46-year-old male, whose symptoms consisted of anxiety, compulsive behavior, depressed mood, irritability, pressured speech, racing thoughts, and paranoia. He was required by his employer to seek psychiatric treatment for erratic behavior at work. Evaluation also revealed premorbid symptoms such as odd beliefs and thinking, suspiciousness, eccentric behavior, ideas of reference, grandiosity, lack of empathy, and exploitative tendencies. He denied drug and alcohol abuse, smoking, and caffeine intake. The patient had been taking fluoxetine 20 mg intermittently for about a year prior to his first office visit. He had never been married and lived by himself. He denied a family history of psychiatric problems. The patient denied a history of medical problems.

Axis II Diagnosis: Schizotypal personality disorder with narcissistic features

Axis I Diagnosis: Bipolar disorder, not otherwise specified obsessive-compulsive features

Current Treatment:
1. lithium (Eskalith CR) 450 mg BID
2. fluoxetine 20 mg AM
3. risperidone 0.5 mg HS
4. psychotherapy

Treatment Course: Risperidone 0.5 mg HS was started at the first visit. Lithium was introduced when the patient was seen two weeks later. The patient was advised to continue fluoxetine at 20 mg AM. Depressive, schizotypal, and hypomanic symptoms showed satisfactory improvement. The lithium level was 0.7 mEq/L. The thyroid profile was normal.

Comments: This patient's symptoms and effective medications can be grouped as follows:

Symptom Group	Medication Class	Specific Medication
Bipolar	mood stabilizer	lithium
Depression, anxiety	antidepressant	fluoxetine
Obsessive-compulsive	antiobsessional	fluoxetine
Schizotypal	antipsychotic	risperidone
Narcissistic/hypomanic	mood stabilizer	lithium

Both symptoms and medications have overlapping features, preventing precise classification. Therefore, the classifications given here are to be seen as an example of organizing clinical material and of selecting medications, rather than as rigid or mutually exclusive entities. For instance, fluoxetine has antidepressant, antianxiety, and antiobsessional effects. Similarly, risperidone has antimanic and antipsychotic properties. Moreover, bipolar symptoms and narcissistic symptoms have some overlapping features and hence could respond to a mood stabilizer.

Case #15

Presenting Symptoms: The patient was a 44-year-old male, brought to the office by his mother. His symptoms consisted of difficulty focusing thoughts, ideas of reference, insomnia, vague and circumstantial thinking, apathy, constricted affect, paranoid ideation, seclusiveness, excessive preoccupation with abstract topics, excessive orderliness, concrete and rigid thinking, and perfectionistic tendencies. The patient's mother reported that most of the above symptoms had been present since early adolescence. the patient denied drug and alcohol abuse, smoking, and caffeine intake. He denied a family history of psychiatric disorders.

Axis II Diagnosis: Schizotypal personality disorder with obsessive-compulsive personality features

Current Treatment:
1. mesoridazine 25 mg HS
2. clomipramine 25 mg HS
3. lorazepam 1 mg HS

(patient noncompliant with psychotherapy)

Treatment Course: Mesoridazine 25 mg HS and lorazepam 1 mg HS were started at the first visit. Schizotypal symptoms improved somewhat. A dosage increase to mesoridazine 50 mg HS would have been beneficial, but the patient did not wish to increase the dose. A switch to risperidone was recommended in early 1994 when it became available, but the patient wanted to continue mesoridazine. Since the obsessive-compulsive personality symptoms persisted, clomipramine 25 mg HS was added, resulting in moderate overall improvement. The patient was able to function as a full-time employee in a semiskilled job after he started the treatment.

Comments: Obsessive-compulsive symptoms are not uncommon in patients with predominantly schizotypal and paranoid personality disorders; hence the treatment frequently consists of a combination of a low dose of an antipsychotic and an SSRI or clomipramine. Treatment using a low dose of an antipsychotic is effective in improving the symptoms of schizotypal personality disorder. Persuasion and active interest by significant others are usually necessary to get people with schizotypal personalities to seek and accept treatment. Since their psychopathology is less severe compared to that of schizophrenics, antipsychotic treatment is successful in most cases. This patient's symptoms and medications may be classified as follows:

Symptom Group	Medication Class	Specific Medication
Schizotypal	antipsychotic	mesoridazine 25 mg HS
Obsessive-compulsive personality	antiobsessional	clomipramine 25 mg HS
Insomnia	sedative-hypnotic	lorazepam 1 mg HS

Case #16

Presenting Symptoms: The patient was a 35-year-old female, who presented with complaints of odd beliefs, depressed mood, disorganized thinking, anxiety, poor concentration, ideas of reference, constricted affect, apathy, mild suspiciousness, insomnia, and anhedonia. These symptoms had been present since her early twenties. She denied drug and alcohol abuse, smoking, and caffeine intake. The patient also denied past psychiatric evaluation or treatment. Her father had a "mental problem" and was institutionalized for many years.

Axis II Diagnosis: Schizotypal personality disorder

Current Treatment:
1. sertraline 100 mg AM
2. risperidone 1.5 mg HS
3. lorazepam 0.5 mg HS PRN insomnia
4. referral for psychotherapy

Treatment Course: The patient was started on risperidone 0.5 mg BID, sertraline 25 mg AM, and lorazepam 0.5 mg HS. She reported mild improvement when seen two weeks later. The dose of sertraline was eventually raised to 100 mg AM and risperidone was increased to 1.5 mg HS with satisfactory improvement in all of the presenting symptoms.

Comments: Diagnostically, this patient could very well be classified as having simple schizophrenia, which is an Axis I diagnosis proposed for further study, and is characterized by (1) prominent negative symptoms; (2) poor interpersonal rapport; and (3) marked decline in occupational or academic functioning, as described in *DSM-IV.* Interestingly, Simple Schizophrenia was an official diagnostic term in the 1970s, but was omitted in *DSM-III-R* and *DSM-IV,* and now is in the process of being resurrected possibly for inclusion in *DSM-V.*

Depressed mood or anxiety are nearly always reported by patients with all psychiatric disorders except while manic, hypomanic, or floridly psychotic. When the depressive and anxiety symptoms are secondary, specific treatment of these symptoms is not necessary, because successful treatment of the primary symptoms will lead to improvement of the secondary symptoms of anxiety and depression. Treatment using a low dose of benzodiazepines can be beneficial during the first one or two weeks if anxiety is prominent, even if the anxiety is thought to be secondary to an underlying psychotic process.

Chapter 5

Antisocial Personality Disorder

DSM-IV diagnostic criteria for antisocial personality disorder are as follows:

DSM-IV *CRITERIA AND SYMPTOM CORRELATES*

A. There is a pervasive pattern of disregard for and violation of the rights of others occurring since age 15 years, as indicated by three (or more) of the following:

1. Failure to conform to social norms with respect to lawful behaviors as indicated by repeatedly performing acts that are grounds for arrest.
2. Deceitfulness, as indicated by repeated lying, use of aliases, or conning others for personal profit or pleasure.
3. Impulsivity or failure to plan ahead.
4. Irritability and aggressiveness, as indicated by repeated physical fights or assaults.
5. Reckless disregard for safety of self or others.
6. Consistent irresponsibility, as indicated by repeated failure to sustain consistent work behavior or honor financial obligations.
7. Lack of remorse, as indicated by being indifferent to or rationalizing having hurt, mistreated, or stolen from another.

B. The individual is at least 18 years of age.

C. There is evidence of conduct disorder with onset before age 15 years.

D. The occurrence of antisocial behavior is not exclusively during the course of schizophrenia or a manic episode.

The potentially treatable symptoms corresponding to *DSM-IV* diagnostic criteria are listed in Table 5.1.

There is no currently available treatment for most of the core symptoms defining antisocial personality disorder. Inclusion of antisocial personality disorder among psychiatric disorders has the unintended effect of "medicalizing" essentially criminal character and conduct the management of which should be the appropriate duty of

TABLE 5.1. Symptom Correlates for Antisocial Personality Disorder

DSM-IV **Criteria**	**Possible Symptom Correlates**
1. Failure to conform to social norms with respect to lawful behaviors as indicated by repeatedly performing acts that are grounds for arrest	criminal behavior (no medical treatment yet available)
2. Deceitfulness, as indicated by repeated use of aliases, or conning others for personal profit or pleasure	exploitative conduct and lying (no medical treatment yet available)
3. Impulsivity or failure to plan ahead	impulsivity
4. Irritability and aggressiveness, as indicated by repeated physical fights or assaults	irritability, anger, hostility
5. Reckless disregard for safety of self or others	possibly related to impulsivity and anger
6. Consistent irresponsibility, as indicated by repeated failure to sustain consistent work behavior or honor financial obligations	irresponsibility (no medical treatment yet available)
7. Lack of remorse, as indicated by being indifferent to or rationalizing having hurt, mistreated, or stolen from another	defective conscience (no medical treatment yet available)

the judiciary system. However, there are aspects of antisocial personality disorder which may respond to treatment. Impulsivity, for example, could be the manifestation of adult attention deficit hyperactivity disorder or hypomanic states of mind. Thus, depending upon the underlying disorder, treatment is possible. Attention deficit hyperactivity disorder could respond to various medications such as bupropion, imipramine, stimulants, clonidine, guanfacine, venlafaxine, or pemoline (Cylert), whereas hypomania can be treated using lithium, carbamazepine, sodium valproate, gabapentin, lamotrigine, verapamil, clonazepam and, as a last resort, using antipsychotics, or using combinations of the above medications. Since an individual with antisocial personality disorder is at high risk for substance abuse, caution should be used in prescribing medications that have abuse or illicit sale potential, such as stimulants or benzodiazepines. Other symptoms that might respond to treatment are irritability and anger, which can respond to serotonergic antidepressants, benzodiazepines, or antipsychotics. Obviously, serotonergic medications are the preferred choice. The use of benzodiazepines or antipsychotics should be attempted only if other treatments fail. Case #17 illustrates the use of an antipsychotic with good results. Serotonergic antidepressants are particularly effective in controlling irritability, anger, and hostility. Patients must be informed in a matter-of-fact way that the treatment, at best, is intended as a trial to give them control over impulsivity, irritability, and anger, and that their criminal behavior, exploitative conduct, and disregard for the rights of others are suggestive of a defect in conscience representing the core symptoms and are not expected to improve. They should be further informed that there are no medical treatments currently available for the latter problems. If the patient is brought by significant others or ordered by the court, he or she should also be informed of the limited expectation of positive results from treatment and of the expectation that criminal conduct is likely to continue at a baseline level. Even with trials on different medications, in the author's experience, the success rate is low. However, there is a minority for whom significant improvement in impulsivity and irritability are evident. Case #18 is an example. Since there is no reliable means to predict the outcome of treatment for a particular individual, the physician should give an empiric trial of treatment for most patients (assuming they will accept it). There may be antisocial personalities without impulsivity or irritability as symptoms; for these patients there would be no treatable symptoms at all. In those cases, obviously, the physician should inform the patient and the concerned family or referral source (with the patient's permission) that medical treatment is not available. Group therapy can be of some help and may be recommended to patients with antisocial personality disorder; however, patients typically are non-compliant unless forced by threats of incarceration or other sanctions. The same is true for compliance with medication treatment.

The physician should exercise caution not to encourage the patient or the legal system to exploit the psychiatric evaluation or treatment by using them as a substitute for legal consequences. It is the defense lawyer's job to get an offender the least punishment by whatever legal means available, including psychiatric evaluation, testimony, and services that, unfortunately, are used frequently and inappropriately to rationalize unlawful behavior, or to avoid punishment.

Since patients with antisocial personality disorder are at high risk for substance abuse, which further exacerbates impulsivity, irritability, and other antisocial behavior, it is important to consider prophylactic use of medications, which can diminish the reinforcement properties of abusive drugs such as alcohol and narcotics. One such medication is naltrexone at 50 mg daily. Since substance abuse is a common problem among patients with emotional disorders, naltrexone should be considered in all patients at risk for substance abuse.

Examples of various combination treatments for certain potentially treatable symptoms in antisocial personality disorder are given below:

1. bupropion 100 mg BID
   valproic acid 250 mg TID
   naltrexone 50 mg HS

   In this combination, bupropion can improve depressive and attention deficit problems, valproic acid can treat hypomania and related impulsivity, and naltrexone can diminish substance abuse tendencies.

2. paroxetine 20 mg AM
   lithium carbonate 300 mg BID-TID

   In this example, paroxetine can treat irritability and anger, and lithium can improve impulsivity.

3. imipramine 100 mg HS
   carbamazepine 200 mg BID

   Imipramine has the potential to improve attention deficit hyperactivity symptoms, impulsivity, dysphoria, irritability, and anger. Carbamazepine can treat hypomanic symptoms as well as aggressive tendencies.

Some symptoms that are part of the antisocial personality disorder criteria and have the potential to be improved with treatment are described above. Obviously, people with antisocial personality disorder, like anyone else, can develop symptoms of depression, panic, psychosis, etc., which should be treated as they emerge. It should be pointed out to patients and concerned individuals (with the patients' permission) that the primary symptoms in antisocial personality disorder cannot be treated medically, that the medical treatment strategies are aimed toward improvement of the limited symptoms, and that the probability of success is dependent upon compliance with treatment and abstinence from substance abuse.

It is an interesting observation that impulsivity, defective learning and uninhibited behavior are characteristics shared by attention deficit hyperactivity disorder and conduct disorder, and that stimulants improve these characteristics. Individuals with antisocial personality disorder also have difficulty learning from negative consequences (and from threats of punishment). Can stimulants improve the learning function in antisocials and thereby make them capable of developing a conscience? Could specific medications be developed to improve learning and to enhance inhibitions among antisocials? Perhaps further research could help synthesize medications to treat the core symptoms of antisocial personality disorder, but there is nothing on the horizon for the near future.

CLINICAL CASES 17 to 19

Case #17

Presenting Symptoms: The patient was a 49-year-old male, with symptoms consisting of homicidal ideation and threats toward his ex-wife, stalking her despite a restraining order, frequent suicidal ideation, deep-seated anger, belief that his wife was responsible for all of his problems, hostility, bitterness, distrust of people, extreme selfishness, depressed mood, violent behavior toward his ex-wife, destruction of his ex-wife's properties (slashing her car tires, placing dead animals in front of her door), lack of remorse, threats to commit suicide if sent to jail, and obsessive-compulsive tendencies. These symptoms at a lower level of severity had been present for many years. This patient's history also suggests the presence of conduct disturbance during his teenage years. He denied drug and alcohol abuse, and caffeine intake. He reported smoking one pack of cigarettes per day. The patient had been taking sertraline 150 mg daily when first seen at my office. He denied any family psychiatric history. His medical history was unremarkable.

Axis II Diagnosis: Antisocial personality disorder with paranoid, narcissistic, and obsessional features

Axis I Diagnosis: Schizoaffective disorder, depressed

Current Treatment:
1. risperidone 2 mg AM and 4 mg HS
2. fluoxetine 40 mg AM
3. psychotherapy

Treatment Course: The patient was hospitalized for ten days and discharged on the above medications in significantly improved condition. He has been compliant with treatment. He was sentenced to jail where he received medications as listed above. He completed his jail term and was released about six months ago. Since his release, he had shown continued compliance and improvement in symptoms such as hostility, paranoia, suicidal thoughts, and obsessive preoccupation with harming his estranged wife.

Comments: When a patient presents with despicable attitudes and behavior, it is almost routine to attribute them to a personality disorder. It is of some concern that despite being involved in the mental health-forensic system for nearly two years, this patient was not given antipsychotic medication. The author's speculation is that a fatalistic attitude emerged among mental health clinicians after someone diagnosed him with a personality disorder. Setting aside the formal diagnosis, an analysis of his behavior and attitudes shows the following:

Symptoms	Medication
Extreme hostility	antipsychotic
Paranoia	antipsychotic
Extreme externalization of blame	antipsychotic
Suicidal thoughts	antidepressant
Obsessive-compulsive symptoms	SSRI or clomipramine
Hypersomnia	stimulating antidepressant
Anger attacks	SSRI

It is evident from a symptom analysis that the combination of an antipsychotic and an SSRI antidepressant should address the major symptoms. Fortunately, risperidone and fluoxetine were effective and well-tolerated by the patient. Medication treatment provides improved internal control in which the patient is deficient without the medication. One of the purposes of psychotherapy with patients who have deficiencies in ego and superego functions is to enhance and strengthen internal controls. The process of psychotherapy works much more efficiently after the medication has prepared the mind to incorporate the insights and to learn. One of the positive effects of the legal sanctions involving external controls such as incarceration, probation, and various disciplinary actions is also to enhance internal control, so that the offending behavior will be inhibited in the future. In essence, the fear of punishment acts as an internal control force. Obviously, medication treatment and psychotherapy are not substitutes for punishment, which serves other functions. Internal controls are primarily a result of learning. For example, a baby does not become civilized unless it is nurtured and taught. Potential for learning is variable. For instance, a patient with attention deficit disorder (ADD) or mental retardation has difficulty learning. In some cases, as in ADD, medication treatment enables patients to learn more effectively. Similarly, when patients are burdened by symptoms, regardless of Axis I or Axis II classification, treatment with medication is almost always beneficial, especially if psychotherapy, which is a form of corrective learning process, is to be maximally exploited. Medication and psychotherapy are complementary, and may even have synergistic effects.

It must be emphasized again that personality disorders, just like any other disorders, should be assessed in terms of specific component symptoms that are then treated using appropriate medications. This is very similar to a skilled psychotherapist understanding the patient's verbalizations in terms of conflicts, defenses, and patterns, and employing specific psychotherapeutic techniques in an organized and disciplined manner to achieve the goals of psychotherapy. Most patients with symptoms will benefit from medication, which, in turn, makes psychotherapy more effective.

Case #18

Presenting Symptoms: The patient was a 25-year-old male, with complaints of depressed mood, hypersomnia, irritability, multiple recurring legal problems, a history of stealing and lying, conduct disorder as a teenager, imprisonment for five months, a recent charge of resisting arrest, frequent fights, irresponsible behavior, impulsivity, poor frustration tolerance, anhedonia, anergia, and feelings of hopelessness. The patient sought psychiatric services at the urging of his defense lawyer. The patient claimed that his attorney advised him that a psychiatric evaluation and treatment could help his legal case. He had a long history of multiple substance abuse during his teens but stopped the abuse several years ago. He reported smoking one pack of cigarettes daily. He denied caffeine intake. His mother had been diagnosed with depression and was taking fluoxetine. The patient was discharged from military service because of insubordination. He denied major medical problems.

Axis II Diagnosis: Antisocial personality disorder

Axis I Diagnosis: Dysthymia
Mild attention deficit disorder (ADD)

Current Treatment:
1. fluoxetine 20 mg AM
2. bupropion 100 mg AM and noon
3. psychotherapy referral

Treatment Course: At the first visit this patient was started on fluoxetine 10 mg AM, and bupropion 100 mg AM with instruction to increase bupropion to 100 mg AM and noon. At the second visit two weeks later, he reported significant improvement in ADD symptoms and hypersomnia, but complained of irritability, depression, and anger; hence, fluoxetine was increased to 20 mg AM. When seen two weeks later, there was further improvement in irritability, depressed mood, and anger.

Comments: Patients with antisocial personality disorder typically do not seek psychiatric help voluntarily. The consequences of their antisocial behavior lead to legal problems, interpersonal problems, and secondary Axis I symptoms such as depression, insomnia, etc. These secondary symptoms and coexisting conditions (dysthymia and ADD, in this case) are amenable to treatment. Most of the core antisocial symptoms such as illegal acts, irresponsibility, lack of remorse, and deceitfulness do not respond to currently available medication treatment. Irritability, impulsivity, and hostility which can be some of the symptoms of antisocial personality disorder, might improve on treatment with antidepressants or a low dose of an antipsychotic.

The patient and his girlfriend (who accompanied him into the office and was present during the sessions) were told that treatment could benefit his depressive and ADD symptoms, but not the core antisocial symptoms.

Good defense lawyers routinely instruct their clients to seek psychiatric treatment and then present the record of psychiatric evaluation and treatment to the court in an attempt to obtain the most favorable judgment for their clients. Who wouldn't get depressed when faced with the possibility of a jail term? Even antisocials become depressed and anxious when they are forced to deal with the consequences of their behavior. Mental health professionals unwittingly facilitate the pattern of exploitation by the antisocial individual when psychiatric rationalization is offered for essentially criminal conduct, thereby making it more difficult for the individual to learn to take responsibility for his/her behavior.

Two classes of antidepressants were employed in the treatment of this patient to address two discrete symptoms that respond preferentially to different antidepressants.

Symptom Groups	Medication
ADD symptoms, hypersomnia	bupropion
Irritability, hostility, impulsivity, depressed mood	fluoxetine

Case #19

Presenting Symptoms: The patient was a 15-year-old male, with symptoms of disobedience, stealing, lying, impulsivity, truancy, frequent violence toward others, anger outbursts, increased irritability, distractibility, poor concentration, disruptive classroom behavior, and moodiness. He was suspended from school on several occasions. The patient's mother–who brought him to the office–provided the clinical information and reported that these behaviors had been getting worse for the past five years. He denied drug and alcohol abuse, and smoking. He also denied previous psychiatric evaluation or treatments. The patient's mother suffered from depression and his father from mood swings. This patient had been living with his mother since age three when his parents divorced.

Current Diagnosis (Axis I): Conduct disorder
Attention deficit disorder (ADD)
Dysthymia

Current Treatment:
1. paroxetine 10 mg AM
2. dextroamphetamine 5 mg AM and 2 PM
3. referral to counselor

Treatment Course: The patient was started on paroxetine 10 mg AM and dextroamphetamine 5 mg AM and at 2 PM at the first visit. Since the patient and his mother reported satisfactory results, the patient is maintained on the above medications.

Comments: Conduct disorders tend to progress to antisocial personality disorder, which is a diagnosis that cannot be given to individuals younger than 18 years old, according to *DSM-IV* criteria. Therefore, a conduct disorder may be considered a childhood form of antisocial personality disorder from a clinical perspective. However, conduct disorder is classified as an Axis I disorder and antisocial personality disorder is classified as an Axis II disorder. Certain symptoms that are features of antisocial personality disorder such as impulsivity, irritability, aggressiveness, anger and hostility might respond to treatment. The core symptoms that define antisocial personality disorder such as criminal conduct, exploitative conduct, irresponsible behavior, and conscious violation of the rights of others (all suggesting defective conscience or "superego") do not currently lend themselves to effective pharmacological treatment.

Frequently symptoms of ADD, oppositional defiant disorder and dysthymia can overlap. At times, effective treatment of the overlapping symptoms can have a beneficial effect on some of the conduct disorder (antisocial) symptoms, as was observed in this case. If the patient only had conduct disorder symptoms, I doubt that the treatment outcome would be as satisfactory.

Chapter 6

Borderline Personality Disorder

Borderline personality disorder is characterized by the following *DSM-IV* criteria.

DSM-IV *CRITERIA AND SYMPTOM CORRELATES*

A pervasive pattern of instability of interpersonal relationships, self-image, and affects, and marked impulsivity beginning by early adulthood and present in a variety of contexts, as indicated by five (or more) of the following:

1. *Frantic efforts to avoid real or imagined abandonment. (Note: Do not include suicidal or self-mutilating behavior covered in Criterion 5.)*
2. *A pattern of unstable and intense interpersonal relationships characterized by alternating between extremes of idealization and devaluation.*
3. *Identity disturbance–markedly and persistently unstable self-image or sense of self.*
4. *Impulsivity in at least two areas that are potentially self-damaging (e.g., spending, sex, substance abuse, reckless driving, binge eating). (Note: Do not include suicidal or self-mutilating behavior covered in Criterion 5.)*
5. *Recurrent suicidal behavior, gestures, or threats, or self-mutilating behavior.*

---

6. *Affective instability due to a marked reactivity of mood (e.g., intense episodic dysphoria, irritability, or anxiety usually lasting a few hours and only rarely more than a few days).*
7. *Chronic feelings of emptiness.*
8. *Inappropriate, intense anger or difficulty controlling anger (e.g., frequent displays of temper, constant anger, recurrent physical fights).*
9. *Transient, stress-related paranoid ideation or severe dissociative symptoms.*

An analysis of symptom correlates reveals that the borderline personality disorder encompasses a variety of symptoms that probably require drugs from different medication classes for optimal response (see Table 6.1). Hypomanic, depressive, anxiety, and psychotic symptoms at varying degrees of severity are seen in individuals with borderline personality disorder. In fact, most of the patients diagnosed by other clinicians as suffering from borderline personality disorder and referred to the author for management or second opinion consultations are frequently found to qualify for one or more of the following diagnoses: schizoaffective disorder–bipolar or depressed type, bipolar disorders, depressive disorders with psychotic features, cyclothymia, adult ADHD, polysubstance abuse, PTSD, and various other personality traits. The author's admitted bias in favor of focusing on symptoms and diagnosing Axis I disorders whenever possible, is evident in the clinical cases that follow. There is considerable range of severity among borderline personality disorder patients. Patients with borderline personality disorder are informally categorized from low functioning to high functioning. Low-functioning borderline personality disorder suggests more severe symptoms and more pronounced dysfunction compared to the higher-functioning patients. Since they present complicated management challenges, and thereby test the clinical skills of mental health staff, there is considerable frustration and ambivalence toward treating a patient with borderline personality features. The extent of countertransference hostility among psychiatric staff toward a patient with borderline personality disorder is such that the word borderline is the equivalent of a psychiatric four-letter word. There is a tendency among mental health professionals to brand a patient as borderline if the

TABLE 6.1. Symptom Correlates for Borderline Personality Disorder

	DSM-IV Criteria	Symptom Correlates
1.	Frantic efforts to avoid real or imagined abandonment	obsessive fear and separation anxiety, rejection sensitivity
2.	A pattern of unstable and intense interpersonal relationships characterized by alternating between extremes of idealization and devaluation	labile affect, mood swings
3.	Identity disturbance—markedly and persistently unstable self-image or sense of self	mild thought disorganization and regression
4.	Impulsivity in at least two areas that are potentially self-damaging (e.g., spending, sex, substance abuse, reckless driving, binge eating)	hypomanic symptoms, impulsivity
5.	Recurrent suicidal behavior, gestures or threats, or self-mutilating behavior	depression, anger, compulsions
6.	Affective instability due to a marked reactivity of mood (e.g., intense episodic dysphoria, irritability, or anxiety usually lasting a few hours and only rarely more than a few days)	rapid mood swings, anxiety
7.	Chronic feelings of emptiness	depression
8.	Inappropriate, intense anger or difficulty controlling anger (e.g., frequent displays of temper, constant anger, recurrent physical flights)	anger, irritability, hostility
9.	Transient, stress-related paranoid ideation or severe dissociative symptoms	paranoia, mild psychotic symptoms (regressive)

patient is hostile, demanding, emotionally needy, uncooperative, moody, irritable, or disruptive, so much so that the word borderline implies "headache" for the treating staff. Unfortunately, there is a myth among many psychiatric staff that borderline personality disorder is not treatable, and that efforts made by the staff are a waste of time. In many instances, mental health professionals give up when one or two medication classes fail to significantly improve the patient's condition. Complex psychopharmacological management is usually required to successfully treat a low-functioning borderline patient. Many psychiatrists are trained to frown upon polypharmacy and hence feel helpless when dealing with a borderline patient. In general polypharmacy is to be avoided if possible, as is true in all areas of medicine. However, the psychiatrist treating a borderline patient must be adept at the rational, artful, and balanced use of polypharmacy with use of medications from three to four different medication classes simultaneously or at various times. In terms of complexity, the medication treatment of a typical borderline personality is second only to a complex schizoaffective disorder, bipolar type, or bipolar disorder. Psychotherapeutic treatment is also similarly complicated. However, stabilization on medication enables patients to benefit significantly from psychotherapy so that rather than being a forum for regression, the patient can be more receptive to learning.

The following classes of medications in Table 6.2 are necessary at some point in the medication treatment of most borderline personality disorders. However in the majority of patients, particularly in moderately severe or severe (low-functioning) borderline personality disorder, a combination involving most of the following classes of medications is necessary for optimal symptom control.

Symptom cluster analysis shows that a borderline patient with a few associated symptoms will need medications from four to six classes of medication, with the possibility of secondary medications such as anticholinergics, H2 blockers, or beta blockers needed to control side effects of the primary medications. Given the significant risk of suicide, estimated at 10 percent among patients with borderline personality disorder, the morbidity and mortality rate approaches that of schizophrenia, bipolar disorder, and major depression, making borderline personality disorder one of the most serious psychiatric

TABLE 6.2. Symptom-Based Medication Guide for Borderline Personality Disorder

Primary Symptom Cluster	Medication Classes Likely to Control the Symptoms
Mood swings, labile affect, rapid cycling, hypomanic symptoms, impulsivity (possible cyclothymia)	mood stabilizers such as lithium carbonate, valproic acid, carbamazepine, gabapentin, verapamil, lamotrigine, or clonazepam
Depression, anger, irritability, impulsivity, hostility, obsessive fear, rejection sensitivity, anxiety, compulsions, self mutilation	serotonergic antidepressants, bupropion, MAOIs, TCAs (adjunctive naltrexone possibly effective for compulsive self-mutilation)
Paranoia, hostility, psychotic regression, mild thought disorganization, irrational thinking	antipsychotics at low doses (for low-functioning patients, clozapine may be effective); risperidone, olanzapine, and sertindole preferred as general purpose first-line antipsychotics
Anxiety symptoms	antianxiety medications at low doses, and/or antidepressants
Associated Symptoms/Disorders	
High risk of substance abuse	naltrexone
Post-traumatic stress disorder	trazodone, busiprone, antianxiety medications, antipsychotics, clonidine
Attention deficit hyperactivity disorder	stimulants, bupropion, TCAs, pemoline
Dissociative symptoms	antipsychotics (low dose)
Irrational hostility	antipsychotics (low dose), risperidone, olanzapine, or sertindole preferred

disorders or among the most life-threatening disorders, deserving aggressive psychiatric management. If mental health professionals made an effort to search for specific treatable symptoms in a patient with borderline personality disorder just as diligently as they do in patients with schizoaffective disorder, major depression, or bipolar disorder, the prevalent derogatory attitudes and ambivalence toward borderline patients would change. This change would benefit patients significantly and enable the mental health professionals to derive the ultimate fulfillment of satisfactorily managing difficult patients. In some cases, the physician needs to know details of specific symptoms in order to choose the most appropriate treatment. An example is the symptom of insomnia. The physician needs to know the specific type of insomnia–initial, middle, or terminal insomnia, each of which has a different medication of choice.

There is no better example than borderline personality disorder to illustrate the concept that it is primarily symptoms, not diagnosis, that determine the choice of medication treatment, though this approach is valid in all diagnoses including major depression, schizoaffective disorder, bipolar disorder, and schizophrenia. Other factors such as medication formulations (PO or IM), the presence of allergies, or cost and family history of medication response are also factors, but the most important determinant of medication choice is the presence or absence of specific symptoms. A diagnosis gives general information that is not sufficient to make optimal medication decisions; hence, it is extremely important to obtain a thorough enumeration of symptoms, regardless of the diagnosis. This is not only true in psychiatry but also in other medical specialties. The physician needs to know the specific symptoms in order to choose various medications and dosages that would yield the most efficient and effective treatment response, particularly in fairly heterogenous conditions such as schizoaffective disorder or borderline personality disorder. Examples of medication regimens are given below.

1. A borderline patient with rapid mood swings, impulsivity, hypomanic symptoms, dysphoria, anger, irritability, paranoia, alcohol abuse, and initial insomnia would need a mood stabilizer that is effective for rapid cycling, an antidepressant, a low dose of an antipsychotic, a fast acting hypnotic, and a medication to aid alcohol treatment.

Example:

valproic acid 250 mg TID
paroxetine 20 mg AM
risperidone 0.5 mg HS
trazodone 50 mg HS PRN insomnia
naltrexone 50 mg with supper

In addition, supportive psychotherapy, and alcohol treatment including Alcoholics Anonymous are necessary at a minimum.

2. A borderline patient with obsessive-compulsive symptoms, anger outbursts, mood swings, irritability, anxiety, depression, and identity disturbance (but no hypomanic or regressive symptoms) could be treated with an antidepressant alone, such as any of the serotonergic antidepressants, nefazodone, venlafaxine, mirtazapine, clomipramine, or bupropion, and supportive psychotherapy.

A heterogenous disorder such as borderline personality disorder can present with such varied symptomatology that each individual patient's specific symptoms determine the selection of specific medications to a greater extent than in many other disorders. For example, even in a broad diagnostic class such as psychosis, the need for an antipsychotic is predictable. Such is not the case with borderline personality disorder, in which a particular patient might partially respond to any one of the major classes of psychiatric medications. Obviously, the realistic goal of treating a borderline personality disorder, or any chronic condition, is to control symptoms significantly to the extent that the person can lead a satisfactory life with medications playing an important part of a multimodal treatment strategy involving psychological, social, rehabilitative, and preventive measures. Generally, medications with addictive potential should be avoided in treating patients with borderline personality disorder. Although the safest antidepressants are the non-TCA and non-MAOI antidepressants, many borderline patients need TCAs or MAOIs for proper symptom resolution.

3. A borderline patient with severe mood swings, impulsivity, aggressive behavior, hypomanic symptoms, and dysphoria could be controlled on a mood stabilizer alone or on a combination of mood stabilizers, along with psychosocial treatment approaches.

4. A borderline patient with regressive behavior, episodic psychosis, paranoia, episodic hypomania, hostility, severe identity conflicts, dissociative episodes, and deteriorated functioning could potentially be treated with a single antipsychotic. Risperidone, olanzapine, and sertindole are preferred as general purpose, first-line antipsychotics. However, the author's experience suggests that most borderline patients need combinations of two or more different classes of medications for optimal control of symptoms. A chronically low-functioning and treatment-resistant borderline patient with predominant psychotic symptoms could respond well to clozapine (although clozapine is not approved by the FDA for treating borderline personality disorder).

TREATING AND WORKING WITH SUICIDAL PATIENTS

Emotionally disordered patients are at risk for self-defeating, actively self-destructive, and in severe cases, suicidal behavior. Suicide attempts occur, despite the best efforts of the clinician and despite compliance by the patient. Clinicians should always keep in mind that a patient who is determined to commit suicide will be successful sooner or later, regardless of the clinician's efforts to prevent it. Psychiatric hospitalization and 24-hour one-to-one supervision are only short-term interventions and are not practical long-term solutions for a patient who is chronically suicidal. It is critical to recognize that a susceptible patient may not be successful even after many serious attempts and that another less fortunate patient may be successful at the very first attempt. There are many external factors which are beyond the clinician's as well as the patient's control that determine whether or not a suicide attempt is successful. Many determined patients are successful in their suicide attempts even when they are in a hospital environment. It is neither practical nor realistic to expect to prevent suicidal behavior, which should be seen as one of the symptoms of a patient's illness and should be aggressively treated. If you suspect suicide potential, the patient and concerned significant others should be told that the patient has suicide potential, that the risk of suicide exists, that the clinician does not have control over the patient's behavior, and that treatment is expected to improve the condition but, as in any field of medicine, there can be no guarantees of successful outcome. They should be told that though practical treatments will be recommended, including hospitalization, ultimately patients have control over their own fates. Only a small minority of suicidal patients have chronic suicidal ideation. Moreover, if a patient reports a decrease in suicidal thoughts, most hospitals consider discontinuation of suicidal precautions (which are not foolproof anyway) and consider discharge. In most cases, even in state hospitals where the stay is typically long-term, unless patients are actively suicidal or self-destructive, they are discharged to their communities. In the majority of patients, suicidal ideation and suicidal behavior are intermittent and largely unpredictable. Therefore, from a practical and rational standpoint, it is neither possible nor humane to hospitalize a patient forever because of high suicide risk. If the patient and significant others are able to understand and accept this risk and the clinician's limitations, such high suicide-risk patients should pose no conflicts for the clinician. If a patient is uncooperative, by repeatedly being noncompliant or by abuse of alcohol or drugs (illicit or prescribed) despite reasonable efforts by the clinician to help the patient, discharge from the office practice should be considered on the grounds that the clinician is unable to help the patient. Many such patients have a deteriorating course and may need involuntary inpatient treatment at times of exacerbation.

A clinician should expect approximately one suicide attempt for every 100 to 200 patients, with successful suicides comprising approximately 15 percent of the attempts. This ratio means that there is a risk of one to two completed suicides for every 500 cases in a psychiatric practice with a mix of outpatient and inpatient practice. The ratio may be higher for physicians who work for the most part in inpatient crisis centers or with high risk groups such as patients with so called "dual diagnoses" (substance abuse and emotional disorder). The ratio should be lower for clinicians who work only in an outpatient setting. It is critical for clinicians to recognize that if they see a large enough number of patients, sooner or later one of them is going to be successful in committing suicide. Suicide attempts cannot be viewed as personal defeats by the clinician. It is imperative to develop a functional professional detachment (which encompasses compassion).

Any misuse of prescribed medications is an abuse, including overdosing on the medications for the purpose of suicide. Although suicidality is a symptom of a patient's illness, and to some extent beyond the patient's volitional control, overdosing on medications suggests noncompliance and exploitation. If overdosing on medications is repeated despite explanation as to the dynamics of overdose as noted above, the clinician is faced with the consideration of whether or not to terminate the patient from his or her care, based on noncompliance and abuse of treatment. Cases 20 through 30 illustrate medication strategies in the treatment of patients with borderline personality disorder, in a range of complexities.

CLINICAL CASES 20 to 30

Case #20

Presenting Symptoms: The patient was a 25-year-old female, with symptoms consisting of depressed mood, frequent crying, anhedonia, frequent suicidal ideation, a history of suicide gestures by cutting her wrist, impulsivity, feelings of emptiness, feelings of hopelessness, emotional instability, anger outbursts including occasional physical fights, paranoia, insomnia, dissociative episodes, perfectionistic tendencies, and nightmares. Some of these symptoms had been present for the past eight to ten years. She denied acute precipitants. She denied drug and alcohol abuse, smoking and caffeine intake. She had had psychotherapy off and on for many years with some improvement which did not persist. She denied a history of major medical problems and a family history of psychiatric disorders.

Axis II Diagnosis: Borderline personality disorder

Axis I Diagnosis: Major depression, severe, recurrent, with mild psychotic features
Dysthymia

Current Treatment:
1. venlafaxine 100 mg TID
2. risperidone 1 mg AM and 3 mg HS
3. clonazepam 0.25 mg TID
4. trazodone 50 mg HS
5. propranolol 20 mg TID
6. psychotherapy

Treatment Course: The patient was initially started on paroxetine, which was gradually increased to 40 mg AM with no improvement in depressive symptoms. She was switched to fluoxetine, which was eventually given at a dose of 60 mg AM. However, fluoxetine had to be discontinued due to restlessness and increased anxiety. Venlafaxine was started at 25 mg TID and slowly raised to the current dose of 100 mg TID. Other medications were added to control associated symptoms, as described next.

Comments: Depression is typically the presenting symptom in patients with borderline personality disorder; hence, an antidepressant is nearly always necessary for the treatment of borderline personality disorder. In addition to improving depressed mood, antidepressants also have the advantage of improving several of the borderline personality disorder symptoms, such as mood irritability, anger attacks, suicidal or self-injurious behavior, and feelings of emptiness. The new generation antidepressants (SSRIs, venlafaxine, mintazapine, and nefazodone) are well suited for the treatment of borderline personality disorder because of their improved safety even in overdose. A combination of medications involving an antidepressant, an antipsychotic, a mood stabilizer, and an antianxiety medication is occasionally necessary for optimal outcome in the treatment of borderline personality disorder. The symptom groups and the medications that were found to be effective for this particular patient are given below.

Symptom Group	Medication Class	Specific Medication
Depressed mood, suicidal ideation, anger outbursts, and emotional instability	antidepressant	venlafaxine
Paranoia, dissociative episodes, impulsivity	antipsychotic	risperidone
Anxiety, mood instability	mood stabilizer	clonazepam
Insomnia	sedative-hypnotic	trazodone
Tremulousness	beta-blocker	propranolol

If impulsivity and mood instability emerge in the future, consideration will be given to adding a mood stabilizer such as lithium, valproate, or carbamazepine. For patients who have considerable anxiety along with mild mood instability, a low dose of clonazepam is a reasonable choice. Clozapine might be an option for low-functioning borderline patients, particularly if dissociative symptoms, impulsivity, intense anger, suicidality, and psychotic symptoms do not respond adequately to first-line antipsychotics such as olanzapine, risperidone, and sertindole.

Case #21

Presenting Symptoms: The patient was a 67-year-old female, with complaints of chronic suicidal ideation, frequent slicing of her wrists in a suicidal gesture, alternating idealization and devaluation of her husband, episodic auditory hallucinations, chronic feelings of guilt, feelings of helplessness, multiple vague fears, frequent crying, disorganized thoughts, excessive dependency on her husband, conflicts with her family of origin, fear of rejection and abandonment, episodes of paranoid ideation, chronic feelings of worthlessness, and chronic emotional instability. Most of the symptoms listed above had been present since early adulthood. Her past psychiatric history is significant for a history of alcoholism and abuse of prescription sedatives. She had had approximately 12 psychiatric hospitalizations. Numerous medications including TCAs, MAOIs, antipsychotics, benzodiazepines, and SSRIs were tried with no sustained improvement. She was at one point kept on alprazolam 2 mg five times a day and on clonazepam 1 mg QID by other physicians. Risperidone was tried, but was not fully effective. Her medical history was significant for chronic obstructive pulmonary disease. She denied a family history of mental disorders.

Axis II Diagnosis: Borderline personality disorder

Axis I Diagnosis: Major depression, severe, with psychotic features
Consider schizoaffective disorder, depressed

Current Treatment:
1. clozapine 50 mg HS
2. venlafaxine 25 mg TID
3. haloperidol 1 mg BID
4. lorazepam 0.5 mg TID PRN for anxiety
5. psychotherapy

Treatment Course: After several hospitalizations and trials on various medication combinations that failed to control the patient's mood instability and suicidal gestures, it was decided to treat her with clozapine. Dizziness prevented increasing the clozapine dose above 50 mg per day. Since depressed mood, anxiety, fear, and hallucinations persisted, venlafaxine, haloperidol, and lorazepam were added. Axis I and Axis II symptoms improved dramatically on the current combination of medications. Clozapine is believed to be the most important medication responsible for the patient's stability.

Comments: Clozapine is effective for the treatment of Axis I disorders having chronic or significant psychotic symptoms. However, it has also been found to be quite effective for the treatment of the mood instability and psychotic symptoms characteristic of low-functioning borderline personality disorder. The more severe the borderline personality disorder, the more relevant clozapine becomes as a primary medication. As is true of most patients treated with clozapine, adjunctive medications are frequently needed for optimal outcome (current formal FDA approval for clozapine is for the management of treatment-resistant schizophrenia).

Case #22

Presenting Symptoms: The patient was a 28-year-old female, with complaints of depressed mood, rage attacks, frequent crying, racing thoughts, pressured speech, suicidal ideation, extreme rapid mood swings, and episodes of agitation. Since adolescence she had experienced violent rages during which she physically attacked her adopted parents (and later her husband), punched doors and walls, and destroyed property. She also had mood instability, identity conflicts, dissociative episodes, and impulsivity. She has a long history of multiple drug abuse including alcohol, cocaine, and marijuana use. She smoked marijuana daily. She was arrested several times for possession of cocaine and for shoplifting. She had made several suicidal gestures by cutting her wrist. She smoked about two packs of cigarettes and drank two to three cups of coffee daily. Since the patient was adopted at birth, family history was unknown. She had been raped at age 14. Medical history is significant for back and neck pain (resulting from a motor vehicle accident) for which she had been taking carisoprodol 300 mg TID.

Axis II Diagnosis: Borderline personality disorder with dependent and antisocial features

Axis I Diagnosis: Bipolar disorder, mixed
Cannabis dependence

Current Treatment:
1. bupropion 100 mg TID
2. trazodone 100 mg HS
3. risperidone 3 mg HS
4. diphenhydramine 100 mg HS

Treatment Course: Her previous psychiatrists and the author tried her on numerous psychotropic medications including a variety of mood stabilizers, antidepressants, and antipsychotics. She was fairly well stabilized on her current medications. She is maintained on these medications while in jail (for violation of probation), and is willing to try clozapine when she is released from jail.

Comments: Our definition of "stability" needs a revision since the advent of clozapine. It has been the experience of the author that clozapine enables most of the complicated and treatment-resistant patients to achieve a higher level of stability than is possible with other currently available medications.

My expectation based on clinical experience is that clozapine will significantly improve this patient's Axis I and Axis II symptoms. A mood stabilizer (excluding carbamazepine, due to its risk of bone marrow suppression) and an antidepressant (preferably an SSRI, but excluding bupropion and clomipramine due to their effects on seizure threshold) are likely to be added to clozapine for optimal control of varied symptoms, if clozapine alone is not sufficient.

Most complicated patients need medications in addition to clozapine to obtain the best outcome in terms of function. The presence of borderline features qualifies the patient to be considered "complicated." After a patient is maintained on an average dose of clozapine (between 200 and 400 mg per day) for a month, other medications are added sequentially as needed, to arrive at the optimal combination of medication.

Case #23

Presenting Symptoms: The patient was a 43-year-old female, with symptoms consisting of depressed mood, anxiety, insomnia, guilt feelings, feelings of hopelessness, suicidal ideation, panic attacks, frequent crying, increased anger, and a history of several suicide attempts. The acute exacerbation was precipitated by a breakup with her boyfriend. Feelings of ambivalence, kleptomania, compulsive spelling and counting, frequent lying, self-mutilation, impulsivity, a tendency to engage in intense but transient heterosexual relationships, unstable mood, and paranoid ideation had been present since late adolescence. She had had several psychiatric hospitalizations in the past, one of which was for abuse of prescription alprazolam. She was convicted twice for shoplifting. Her three children are in the custody of their father because she had been unable to take care of them. She denied abuse of illicit drugs or alcohol. She also denied smoking or caffeine intake. She denied any family history of emotional disorders. Her medical history is positive for hysterectomy and hypothyroidism. She is taking estrogen and levothyroxine 0.1 mg daily.

Axis II Diagnosis:	Borderline personality disorder
Axis I Diagnosis:	Major depression, severe, recurrent, with mild psychotic features Obsessive-compulsive disorder Kleptomania
Current Treatment:	1. clozapine 50 mg AM and 100 mg HS 2. fluoxetine 40 mg AM 3. psychotherapy

Treatment Course: Various medications including risperidone, Triavil, thioridazine, thiothixene, haloperidol, lithium, divalproex sodium, carbamazepine, phenelzine, tranylcypromine, and various TCAs and SSRIs in different combinations were tried, with only marginal benefit. Relatively improved stability was obtained after starting clozapine. Both Axis I and Axis II symptoms showed improvement.

Comments: There was no doubt that clozapine had a beneficial effect on symptoms that were attributable to borderline personality disorder. The possibility that improvement of the personality disorder symptoms was due to a nonspecific sedative effect of clozapine is unlikely because similarly sedating medications such as thioridazine, Triavil, and combinations of high-potency antipsychotics and benzodiazepines failed to produce such a noticeable effect on the personality disorder symptoms.

Case #24

Presenting Symptoms: The patient was a 38-year-old female, with complaints of mood swings, depressed mood, crying episodes, self-mutilating behavior, brief psychotic episodes, episodes of manic behavior, impulsivity, dissociative episodes, numerous suicide attempts, identity confusion, strong ambivalent feelings toward her husband, and a pattern of episodic self-destructive behavior. The instability of emotions, ambivalence toward significant others, and self-destructive tendencies had been present since early adolescence. She had had numerous psychiatric hospitalizations beginning with her first suicide attempt by overdose at age 15. She had tried all classes of psychotropic medications, including MAOIs, antipsychotics, and mood stabilizers. The patient had a history of binge drinking and episodic drug abuse. She denied smoking and caffeine intake. The patient's father was diagnosed with schizophrenia and alcoholism and committed suicide when the patient was 20 years old. One of the patient's brothers was an alcoholic. Her medical history is significant for migraine headaches.

Axis II Diagnosis: Borderline personality disorder

Axis I Diagnosis: Schizoaffective disorder, bipolar type

Current Treatment:
1. clozapine 200 mg HS
2. paroxetine 20 mg AM
3. lithium (Eskalith CR) 225 mg AM and 450 mg HS
4. continue psychotherapy

Treatment Course: This patient has had a most complicated treatment course over the last three years, with multiple psychiatric hospitalizations, exacerbations, and numerous medication trials. She was tried on a variety of medications including lithium, valproic acid, carbamazepine, risperidone, thioridazine, haloperidol, various TCAs, SSRIs, and phenelzine. Eventually, the patient stabilized well on the medication combination listed above.

Comments: Low-functioning borderline personality disorder patients typically have a major Axis I diagnosis such as schizoaffective disorder, bipolar disorder, or one of the mood disorders. An interesting observation is that with appropriate medication, the treatment suppresses the symptoms attributed to the personality disorder. For instance, the patient's symptoms may be categorized as Axis I and Axis II symptoms as follows. Some overlap is inevitable.

Axis I Symptoms	Axis II Symptoms
depressed mood	self-mutilation
crying episodes	identity confusion
mood swings	ambivalence
suicide attempts	impulsivity
manic behavior	dissociative episodes
impulsivity	self-destructive behavior
psychotic episodes	fluctuating attachments

Her current treatment resulted in significant improvement in both Axis I and Axis II symptoms. The author believes that clozapine is responsible for much of the stability and that clozapine has been uniquely effective. Her stability cannot be attributed primarily to lithium, paroxetine, and alprazolam because she had had these medications (and other complex combinations including other antipsychotics) in the past, with no significant improvement.

Clozapine is an option to be considered particularly in low-functioning borderline personality disorder patients who cannot be stabilized on other medications or combinations of medications, especially if psychotic, dissociative, or other regressive symptoms are chronically present.

It is also the author's opinion, based on practice experience, that borderline personality disorder patients ultimately need two or three different classes of medications even when they are on clozapine. Typically, an antidepressant and a mood stabilizer are necessary; often a low dose of benzodiazepines or naltrexone (if substance abuse has been a problem) is beneficial. In some patients with borderline personality disorder, the stabilization induced by clozapine can be dramatic. Refer to the section on clozapine (Chapter 15) for detailed practical information related to the use of clozapine.

Case #25

Presenting Symptoms: The patient was a 40-year-old female, with complaints of chronically depressed mood, anxiety, insomnia, racing thoughts, episodes of confusion and thought disorganization, memory loss for discrete periods of time, irritability, impulsivity, panic attacks, a history of several suicide attempts by cutting her wrist, feelings of hopelessness, compulsive counting, an obsessive preoccupation with self-mutilation, episodes of vague auditory hallucinations, extreme mood swings, a history of prescription benzodiazepine abuse, and anhedonia. She denied any recent drug and alcohol abuse. She smoked one-half pack of cigarettes per day. She denied caffeine intake.

Her past psychiatric history was significant for approximately ten psychiatric hospitalizations. She had been tried on nearly all antipsychotics, antidepressants, benzodiazepines, as well as lithium, carbamazepine, and valproic acid. Previous psychiatric diagnoses by different psychiatrists were:

Borderline personality disorder
Multiple personality disorder
Bipolar disorder
Temporal lobe epilepsy
Cyclothymia
Schizoaffective disorder
Acute psychotic episode
Schizophrenia, chronic undifferentiated type
Major depression, severe, with psychotic features
Adjustment disorder with depressed mood
Panic disorder
Personality disorder, NOS

She had a history of being severely physically and emotionally abused as a child. She was a college graduate and had a teacher's certificate. She lived in a half-way house at the time of the initial evaluation.

The patient's father suffered from depression. Her medical history is significant for reflux esophagitis and migraine headaches. Hyperventilation EEG showed intermittent activity from the frontal regions, suggesting a suspicion of a partial complex seizure disorder. She was given carbamazepine for three months in 1989, but had stopped because of an exacerbation of her headaches. Valproic acid was tried in 1993, and was discontinued due to abdominal pain, nausea, and vomiting. She did not feel that either carbamazepine or valproic acid were of any help. Nonpsychiatric medications included omeprazole 20 mg AM, metoclopramide 5 mg QID, conjugated estrogen, and medroxyprogesterone.

Axis II Diagnosis: Borderline personality disorder

Axis I Diagnosis: Schizoaffective disorder, depressed
Obsessive-compulsive disorder
Consider multiple personality disorder

Current Treatment:
1. clomipramine 75 mg HS
2. chlorpromazine 25 mg QID
3. risperidone 2 mg HS
4. benztropine 0.5 mg BID
5. temazepam 15 mg HS
6. trazodone 100 mg HS
7. weekly psychotherapy by a psychologist

Treatment Course: Various medications, including carbamazepine, valproic acid, and all available selective serotonin reuptake inhibitors (SSRIs) were tried under my care, with no success. Propranolol LA 80 mg was tried intermittently to treat migraine headaches and akathisia. Buspirone was started adjunctively, but was not helpful. Urecholine 25 mg had to be occasionally used for urinary hesitation caused by the anticholinergic effects of the medications. Chlorpromazine and risperidone were tried alone and in various dosage combinations until the most effective doses were found. She has been able to stay out of the hospital now for one and one-half years, which is the longest hospital-free interval since her psychiatric illness began in her late twenties. She is seen in the office once every four months. She sees a psychologist once every week.

Comments: Complicated, chronic and severely ill patients with mood symptoms typically have multiple psychiatric diagnoses. A patient's major problem can be described in one or two words using a standardized diagnosis. As emphasized in this text, the clinician needs to focus on the patient's specific symptoms in order to choose medications and other treatments. This principle is even more true when dealing with patients having complex psychiatric problems. Diagnoses, including the various personality disorders, have to be translated and understood in terms of component symptoms so that effective treatment may begin. All of the diagnoses for this patient, given by other psychiatrists, were probably reasonable at the time they were made. By the same token, another psychiatrist could justifiably arrive at a diagnosis different from my current diagnosis. Such diagnostic variability is common when dealing with patients as complex this one.

Borderline personality disorder is often used as a pejorative and hostile term for patients who are not responding to treatment and who have difficult temperaments. Many patients with manic, hypomanic, psychotic, and depressive characteristics are agitated, hostile, needy, angry, impulsive, intrusive, labile, ambivalent, self-destructive, impatient, hyperactive, manipulative, defiant, threatening, and accusatory during the acute phases of their illness and when their symptoms are not properly controlled. These symptoms can be easily interpreted as indicative of a personality disorder, usually that of a borderline personality disorder. There are many instances that I can recall when successful medication treatment completely resolved the so-called "personality disorder."

For purposes of pharmacological treatment, dissociative symptoms probably should be considered a form of a minipsychotic episode, and as such might effectively be treated using low doses of an antipsychotic medication. Fortunately, the psychopharmacologist only has to deal with one body, regardless of the number of personalities, all of which are affected by the same medication; whereas for the psychotherapist, the number and prominence of various personalities are important considerations in conducting therapy. Symptoms, if they are dysfunctional and treatable, should be treated irrespective of which personality manifested the symptoms. Careful and thorough evaluation of patients diagnosed as suffering from multiple personality disorder will usually reveal varying numbers of symptoms from the mood and psychotic spectrums of disorders.

The need for a combination of two or more antipsychotics on a fairly long-term schedule is extremely rare. In the acute treatment period, it is fairly common to use two antipsychotics. For example, when switching from a traditional antipsychotic to clozapine or risperidone, the old antipsychotic is tapered off, while the dose of the new antipsychotic is increased gradually. Another example is that of the patient who becomes acutely agitated while being introduced to an antipsychotic which does not have a parenteral form. In the latter case, another antipsychotic that is available in parenteral form is used on a PRN basis. Yet another example is a patient who responds exceptionally well to a low-potency antipsychotic in some respects such as control of agitation or insomnia, but is unable to tolerate a higher dose to control delusions or hallucinations; hence the patient needs another antipsychotic, usually a high-potency antipsychotic that is better tolerated and is effective for the latter symptoms. An example is the combination of clozapine and risperidone or haloperidol. There are other rare clinical situations in which a combination of two antipsychotics is reasonable. I can remember only one other case among more than 800 patients on antipsychotics who needed two traditional antipsychotics for optimal maintenance treatment, apart from combinations involving clozapine and risperidone.

It is usually unnecessary to give anticholinergic medication while the patient is on a low-potency antipsychotic or sedating tricyclic antidepressants (TCAs) that have inherent anticholinergic effects. There is a risk of anticholinergic excess, leading to central anticholinergic syndrome in which one or more highly anticholinergic medications are used, particularly in cases of high doses used in elderly patients. However, there are some patients who benefit from additional anticholinergic medication, despite being on low-potency antipsychotics.

When this patient has another relapse necessitating hospitalization, consideration will be given to a trial of clozapine which, if effective, can probably supplant the need for most of her current psychotropic medications.*

Case #26

Presenting Symptoms: The patient was a 30-year-old female with complaints of depressed mood, chronic feelings of emptiness, anger attacks, extreme mood swings, irritability, insomnia, feelings of hopelessness, excessive dependency on her boyfriend and her mother, scattered thinking, crying episodes, impulsivity, frequent suicidal ideation without intent or plan, episodes of hypomania, and anhedonia. She had a history of several suicide gestures by cutting her wrists. The patient reported that she had been moody and depressed since age 15. Recent stressors included conflicts with her family and her boyfriend. She had a past history of alcohol dependence, but denied any current drug or alcohol abuse. She smoked one pack of cigarettes per day. She denied caffeine intake. The patient was on alprazolam 0.5 mg TID when first seen in my office. She had had one hospitalization at which time she was started on lithium, which she discontinued soon after discharge. Her mother and sister have a history of depression.

Axis II Diagnosis: Borderline personality disorder with dependent and histrionic features

Axis I Diagnosis: Bipolar disorder, NOS
Consider cyclothymia

Current Treatment:
1. Eskalith CR 225 mg AM and 450 mg HS
2. sertraline 50 mg AM
3. trazodone 50 mg HS
4. risperidone 1 mg HS
5. propranolol long-acting 60 mg AM
6. levothyroxine 0.075 mg AM
7. referral for psychotherapy

*Subsequent to the preparation of the galley pages for this book, when it was too late for major rewriting of the case, the patient suffered another relapse and had to be hospitalized. She is now functioning well on just two medications: clozapine 200 mg HS, and fluoxetine 40 mg AM.

Treatment Course: The patient was started on Eskalith CR 450 mg BID, fluoxetine 20 mg AM, and trazodone 50 mg HS, while alprazolam was gradually tapered off over a period of three weeks. The patient complained of restlessness and agitation after about ten days of starting fluoxetine so it was then discontinued. She was switched to sertraline, which was well tolerated. The patient revealed that she has had thoughts of harming people, extreme hostility toward people, had attacked her boyfriend on several occasions, and had had episodes of depersonalization. She was tried on carbamazepine, which was not effective. Perphenazine 4 mg HS controlled the above symptoms effectively. When risperidone became available, she was switched to risperidone 2 mg HS, and eventually decreased to her current dose of 1 mg HS. Lithium caused hypothyroidism which was treated using levothyroxine 0.075 mg AM. She complained of fine tremors of her fingers, thought to be induced by lithium. Propranolol improved the tremors. TSH has been within normal limits at 1.91 mciu/mL. The patient is seen once every four months for medication management.

Comments: It is difficult to sort out the precise diagnosis amid mild forms of bipolar disorder, cyclothymia, and personality disorder with borderline, narcissistic, and histrionic features. Fortunately for the practicing physician, the precise diagnosis is not as important as eliciting or identifying symptoms that help to select the effective medications. For this particular patient, the author is still not certain of the diagnosis, despite treating the patient for more than three years. Regardless of the true diagnosis, it is clear that the present medications are effective, as evidenced by the patient's emotional stability which, according to her, is currently at its best over the last 10 to 15 years. She has been satisfied with her improvement to such an extent that she wants to stay on this combination of medications indefinitely. Note that none of the medications have common abuse potential or cause physiological dependence.

Case #27

Presenting Symptoms: The patient was a 40-year-old female with complaints of racing thoughts, pressured speech, irritability, mood swings, episodes of depressed mood, anger attacks, violent episodes, hypomanic episodes, hyperphagia, anxiety, a history of several suicide gestures and attempts by overdose and by self-mutilation, insomnia, and a past history of alcohol and cocaine abuse that reportedly ended three years ago. She denied current drug or alcohol abuse and smoking. She drank one to two cups of coffee daily. The patient had had two psychiatric hospitalizations previously, the last hospitalization being three years ago. She was on clonazepam 0.5 mg QID, carbamazepine 400 mg po BID, and sertraline 50 mg AM when seen at my office. The patient reported that her father had fits of anger. Her medical history is significant for motor vehicle accidents in 1987 and 1989 in which she had suffered a closed head injury resulting in concussion. Most of her psychiatric problems apparently predated her head injury.

Axis II Diagnosis: Borderline personality disorder

Axis I Diagnosis: Bipolar disorder, NOS
Consider mood disorder due to head injury

Current Treatment:
1. divalproex sodium 250 mg BID
2. Eskalith CR 450 mg HS
3. clonazepam 0.5 mg TID
4. risperidone 1 mg HS
5. trazodone 200 mg HS
6. referral for psychotherapy

Treatment Course: Since the patient was still symptomatic on the medications she was taking at the time of her first visit at my office, medications were changed to divalproex sodium, lithium, and trazodone while maintaining the patient on clonazepam 0.5 mg QID. Her lithium level on the above dose was found to be 0.4 mEq/L, and valproic acid level was 32 ng/mL. Mood swings, racing thoughts, and pressured speech have been well-controlled on divalproex sodium and lithium. During the course of treatment, the patient revealed that she had paranoid ideation for many years. Risperidone 0.5 mg improved the paranoia somewhat, but an increase to 1 mg almost completely treated the paranoia. The patient has been functioning well on the present combination of medications for more than a year.

Comments: One of the goals of pharmacologic treatment is to control discrete symptoms, using the lowest dose of medication. One of the advantages of combination treatment is that low doses of various medications enable optimal control of a variety of symptoms. Another goal of treatment is to treat the symptoms, using the least number of medications. However, in treating disparate symptoms, different medications are both desirable and necessary. The dosages of divalproex sodium and lithium are kept low as indicated by low serum levels. Clinical response is much more important than rigid adherence to obtaining predetermined target serum levels in most cases. Generally, in maintenance treatment, low dosages can be used successfully, thereby minimizing side effects. Most patients with a chronic bipolar disorder require lithium and/or either valproic acid, carbamazepine, gabapentin, or lamotrigine for effective control of mood swings. Since there is an overlap between symptoms of bipolar disorder and borderline personality disorder, mood stabilizers can be used for the treatment of borderline personality disorder with predominant mood symptoms. This patient is currently on the greatest number of medications that she has ever been at one time, but she is also the most functional and the most stable that she has ever been in her adult life, as is evidenced by her continued stability and satisfactory performance in college. Balanced, disciplined, rational, and symptom-focused combination treatment is not only safe and effective, but also enables patients to function at their highest potential.

Case #28

Presenting Symptoms: The patient was a 15-year-old female, with complaints of behavior problems, distractibility, restlessness, extreme mood swings, promiscuity, truancy, impulsivity, anger outbursts, racing thoughts, depressed mood, insomnia, disorganized thoughts, anorexia, anhedonia, a history of suicide gestures, and suicidal ideation without intent or plan. She denied any acute precipitants. She admitted to episodic abuse of alcohol, cocaine, and marijuana. She smoked one-half pack of cigarettes per day. Prior to being seen at my office, this patient had been tried on fluoxetine, hydroxyzine, sertraline, risperidone, stimulants, desipramine, trazodone, divalproex sodium, various antipsychotics, lithium, and carbamazepine. She had several psychiatric hospitalizations, and had been expelled from school for behavior problems. The patient's mother had severe mental illness and the patient was being raised by her grandmother. Her aunt has a diagnosis of schizophrenia. The patient denied any major medical problems.

Axis II Diagnosis:	Borderline personality disorder
Axis I Diagnosis:	Bipolar disorder, NOS Conduct disorder Polysubstance abuse Consider attention deficit disorder (ADD) Consider schizoaffective disorder, bipolar type
Current Treatment:	1. Depakote sprinkle capsule 250 mg BID and 500 mg HS 2. fluoxetine 20 mg AM 3. Triavil 2/25 HS 4. clonidine 0.1 mg BID 5. ranitidine 150 mg HS 6. referral for psychotherapy

Treatment Course: Various medications, including methylphenidate, bupropion, paroxetine, and imipramine were ineffective. The addition of Triavil and clonidine significantly improved restlessness, distractibility, and impulsivity. Ranitidine was added to control treatment-emergent dyspepsia. The patient has shown significant improvement compared to her baseline, but is still emotionally fragile. If this combination is not effective in the future, a trial on clozapine will be considered.

Comments: Without aggressive outpatient medication management, this patient's behavior and emotional functioning would be likely to deteriorate to the point of needing long-term hospitalization.

Behavioral symptoms in an adolescent are likely to be attributed to conduct disorder or a personality disorder. However, symptoms of bipolar disorder in an adolescent are not well-formed or "mature." Therefore, typical symptoms of mania or depression seen in adults are not always applicable to adolescents. Psychiatric manifestations of mood disorders in adolescents consist of behavioral symptoms for the most part. Aggressive outpatient medication treatment should be pursued for adolescents presenting with what appear to be conduct disorders, personality disorders, or other behavioral problems. Inpatient hospitalization can be prevented or the frequency reduced when symptom-focused medication treatment is provided, just as with adults.

The addition of clonidine significantly improved concentration, distractibility, and restlessness in this patient, whereas stimulants and bupropion were not effective. Even for a complex, seemingly treatment-resistant case, diligent efforts by the physician in attempting different medications and combinations, and cooperation by the patient will result in the eventual identification of medications that are helpful to the patient.

This patient's personality disorder symptoms also showed substantial improvement. Impulsivity, drug abuse, disobedience, sexual promiscuity, truancy, suicidality, anger, and mood instability improved significantly. Since borderline personality disorder encompasses a broad spectrum of disparate symptoms, optimal treatment typically requires a combination of medication to treat the discrete symptoms, as summarized below.

Symptoms	Medication
Depression	antidepressant
Mood swings	mood stabilizer
Anxiety	antianxiety and/or antidepressant
Psychosis (mild, transient)	antipsychotic
Impulsivity, ADD symptoms	stimulants and/or antidepressants

Case #29

Presenting Symptoms: The patient was a 34-year-old female, with complaints of depressed mood, suicidal ideation, history of numerous suicidal attempts by overdosing and cutting her wrists, paranoia, anger, hostility, social withdrawal, extreme ambivalence, severe insomnia (a total sleep duration of less than two hours per day, according to the patient's estimate, verified by her husband), physical violence toward her husband, anger outbursts, and labile affect. She denied drug and alcohol abuse, smoking, and caffeine intake. The patient's father and brother reportedly were alcoholics and had suffered from "nervous breakdowns." Her medical history was significant for hypertension, migraine headaches, and peptic ulcer. She had been taking enalapril, atenolol, ranitidine, and sumatriptan SC.

The patient has a long psychiatric history beginning in 1980 when she was first hospitalized for depression. Since then, she has had approximately 65 (sixty-five) psychiatric hospitalizations, many of which were involuntary. Most voluntary hospitalizations were of one to three days duration because typically the patient left against medical advice several days after signing herself in. Since psychiatrists and psychiatric hospitals in her city refused to treat her, her husband had to bring her to another city (a two hour drive) to find psychiatrists and psychiatric hospitals which, unaware of her history, would agree to treat her. Finally, the new psychiatric hospital staff refused to readmit her for treatment because of their frustration in dealing with her (despite her having adequate private insurance coverage). Her local psychiatrist also refused to continue treating her after she became violent in his office. She has had various diagnoses in the past, including borderline personality disorder, schizoaffective disorder, personality disorder NOS, and depression. Some of her previous psychiatrists and most nursing staff describe her simply as "Borderline." She had been tried on nearly all psychiatric medications, including lithium, valproate, carbamazepine, desipramine, amitriptyline, nortriptyline, imipramine, doxepin, amoxapine, trazodone, bupropion, fluoxetine, sertraline, venlafaxine, phenelzine, tranylcypromine, isocarboxazid (no longer available), haloperidol, fluphenazine, chlorpromazine, thioridazine, thiothixene, trifluoperazine, loxapine, chlordiazepoxide, diazepam, clonazepam, alprazolam, triazolam, and zolpidem. At the time she was first seen in my office, her medications and dosages as prescribed by her previous psychiatrist were:

phenelzine 45 mg AM, 45 mg noon, 30 mg PM
(total 120 mg daily)
loxapine 75 mg daily
benztropine 2 mg TID
alprazolam 2 mg QID

Axis II Diagnosis: Borderline personality disorder

Axis I Diagnosis: Schizoaffective disorder, depressed

Current Treatment:
1. clozapine 100 mg BID and 400 mg HS
2. paroxetine 20 mg AM
3. diazepam 10 mg HS
4. Depakote sprinkle capsule 250 mg TID
5. Risperidone 2 mg HS
6. continue psychotherapy

Treatment Course: The patient was first seen in my office with her husband. Her complete history was reviewed in detail, and the patient was evaluated. They were advised that I would provide psychiatric services as long as she was compliant with treatment recommendations and that noncompliance of a significant nature would result in immediate termination. The first recommendation was to electively and voluntarily hospitalize the patient with a specific plan of trying clozapine. The risks and benefits of clozapine treatment were discussed. They were told to think about the recommendations and to call me when she was ready for hospitalization. She was advised to seek the services of another psychiatrist if she decided not to be hospitalized for a trial of clozapine. Her husband called within a week, consenting to hospitalization, which was arranged the same day. All psychiatric medications that she had been on were discontinued. Clozapine was started, according to Sandoz protocol, as reproduced in Chapter 15. Supplemental haloperidol was given during the first seven days to control agitation. Phenobarbital on a tapering schedule was given for ten days to treat alprazolam withdrawal. The first seven days of hospitalization were very stormy, with frequent use of seclusion and restraints, use of IM haloperidol and lorazepam on many occasions, and frequent threats by the patient to leave AMA. Divalproex sodium was added for seizure prophylaxis. Paroxetine improved depressive symptoms. Supplemental risperidone at 2 mg HS controlled breakthrough-positive symptoms not controlled by clozapine. A long-acting sedative such as diazepam was chosen to treat insomnia and to provide possible additional seizure protection. The clozapine level was 532 ng/ml. Her GAF score during the past year and at admission was estimated at 35. At the time of discharge it was 55. If treatment continues to go well, it is expected that she will show further slow and gradual improvement.

Comments: Difficult and complex patients are often labeled "borderline" by mental health professionals. Even when the patient actually has borderline personality disorder, there nearly always coexists Axis I diagnoses that are treatable. It is frequently found that when the Axis I disorder is effectively managed, the personality disorder symptoms subside to a degree that they become dormant. I believe such is the case with this patient. She has not had a hospitalization in the last two years, which is remarkable, given her history of a hospitalization every one to two months. It is too early to conclude that her recovery is long-term, but the preliminary indications from reports by her, her husband, and her therapist are that she is functioning better now than she has been in the last 15 years.

A warning by the clinician that the patient will be terminated for noncompliance should not routinely be given to patients. Noncompliance should be addressed if it becomes a problem in the course of treatment. It is understood and expected that patients will be compliant. In fact, a preemptive warning of termination for noncompliance with no provocation can suggest hostility or an antagonistic attitude on the part of the clinician. However, for certain patients with severe personality disorders and/or substance abuse in whom noncompliance has been a problem in the past, an initial warning may be necessary and therapeutic. Such an approach gives the clinician better control over the management of the patient. If the patient becomes noncompliant with significant aspects of treatment, the clinician will have no choice but to terminate treatment of the patient, because continuation of treatment in the face of noncompliance leads to further loss of control of the treatment process. When the threat is promptly carried out, the patient is more likely to be compliant with the next clinician. If noncompliance is a major concern based on the patient's past psychiatric history, it may be beneficial for the patient to be told that noncompliance is expected and that the patient will be terminated so that hopefully there will be improved compliance with the next clinician. This could have a paradoxical effect, in that it can serve much like a psychological "vaccination" and possibly forestall noncompliance. There are many variations of this technique, depending upon the unique clinical situation. Such techniques are part of the general clinical skills necessary to be an effective clinician.

Monoamine oxidase inhibitors (MAOIs) should only be abruptly discontinued if the clinician is prepared to treat the withdrawal symptoms, consisting of anxiety, insomnia, nightmares, vivid dreams, and agitation. In rare cases, even transient psychosis and delirium can result. MAOIs may be tapered off over a period of seven days to minimize any withdrawal symptoms. This patient was taking phenelzine 120 mg, which is significantly higher than the maximum recommended dose of 90 mg per day; hence, withdrawal symptoms were expected in this patient. However, for clinical reasons, it was decided to stop phenelzine abruptly and to manage the withdrawal symptoms that were controlled with phenobarbital, haloperidol, and clozapine, which the patient was taking for other purposes.

The seizure risk on clozapine above 500 mg daily is estimated at 5 to 6 percent, which is substantial. Therefore, seizure prophylaxis using valproate, gabapentin, or lamotrigine should be considered in patients receiving clozapine at or above 500 mg daily. My preference is valproate because of its mood-stabilizing effects, which may be considered a bonus. Of all of the valproate preparations, Depakote sprinkle capsule is the least irritating to the gastrointestinal tract. Since this patient had peptic ulcer, it was necessary to choose a medication form that was unlikely to exacerbate gastrointestinal symptoms.

If clozapine has to be discontinued for some reason, assuming the patient remains compliant, other options that may be considered for this patient are risperidone, olanzaprine, sertindole, clomipramine, nefazodone or electroconvulsive therapy (ECT), which have never been tried. Occasionally it is necessary to add high-potency antipsychotics such as risperidone, haloperidol, or thiothixene for control of breakthrough-positive symptoms in a patient receiving clozapine.

This patient presents a chronic suicidal risk. It is critical not to minimize the suicidal risk simply because the patient has not been "successful" despite numerous attempts. It is my hope that this patient will continue to be unsuccessful should she attempt suicide again. It is emotionally stressful for a clinician to work with a chronically suicidal patient unless the clinician is able to assume a professional attitude and is able to use a mild level of defenses such as intellectualization, rationalization, and isolation of affect when a patient is successful in committing suicide. The clinician must accept the reality that determined patients will attempt to commit suicide or homicide or engage in other acts of violence to themselves or others, despite the best efforts of the clinician. Long-term commitment in psychiatric units, 24-hour observations, and no-suicide contracts are neither practical nor effective if a patient is sufficiently determined. Most institutions do not keep patients long-term, even if the clinician is successful in getting the patient admitted with a court order. I have had the experience over the years of sending some of the most self-destructive and dangerous patients to state psychiatric hospitals only to discover that at least some of them were discharged to their communities after several weeks or months. The reality, therefore, is that there is no such thing as permanent hospitalization even for the most chronically suicidal patient. Ongoing 24-hour observation and supervision is obviously impossible. No-suicide contracts will not prevent a truly suicidal or homicidal patient from acting on thoughts or impulses. The clinician's goal should be to help the patient overcome those thoughts and prolong life. Any physician or therapist working with severely emotionally disordered patients will, sooner or later, have to deal with a patient suicide or suicide attempt, and will, on rare occasions, deal with a patient who has attempted or committed homicide. Suicide and homicide, or attempts thereof, are risks associated with severe mental disorders, just as sudden death is a risk associated with severe cardiovascular disease. The clinician's task is to recognize the risk, if recognizable, and to manage the patient in order to reduce the risk, using available and practical clinical techniques. Just as prolonging the life of a patient with severe cardiovascular disease is considered a medical success, in psychiatry it should be considered a success if, due to treatment, the patient lives longer or commits or attempts to commit suicide or homicide later than would be the case without treatment. In dealing with such patients my approach, in addition to providing aggressive treatment in the office or hospital, has been to advise the patient and significant others of chronic risks, practical options, absence of any guarantee of success, and of my plan to do what is practical to attempt to help the patient. With some severely disordered patients, the expectation should be that of palliative rather than curative treatment because the risk of suicide or destructive behavior is so high and chronic that the question is, more appropriately, *when* rather than *if* the behavior will be manifested. When patients drink alcohol or abuse drugs, such behaviors become even less predictable.

Despite the true lack of control over patients' behavior, the clinician must not be indifferent when treating a dangerous patient. The clinician has the responsibility to do a reasonable clinical evaluation, recognize risks suggested by the clinical evaluation, and to offer treatment, if indicated. If a patient reports suicidal thoughts, the clinician must take this disclosure seriously and offer appropriate treatment. On the other hand, if the patient denies any suicidal or homicidal ideation during the clinical evaluation but commits suicide on the way home from the clinician's office, there is simply nothing that the clinician could have done. Another scenario exists when a patient admits to suicidal or homicidal thoughts but denies any intent or plan, agrees to seek help if intent or plan develop, assures the clinician that he or she will not act on the thoughts, and agrees to follow treatment recommendations. Should this patient commit suicide in the near future, there, again, is nothing the clinician could have done to intervene. If a clinician insists on hospitalizing or involuntarily committing every patient with suicidal or homicidal thoughts, approximately 75 percent of the patients in every mental health clinician's practice would end up in the hospital. All clinicians will agree that patients having suicidal or homicidal intent or plan need inpatient treatment or some other immediate intervention to protect themselves or others. Patients experiencing suicidal or homicidal ideation clearly need aggressive treatment, but may or may not need inpatient treatment, depending on numerous other factors.

Case #30

Presenting Symptoms: The patient was a 42-year-old female, whose symptoms consisted of depressed mood, insomnia, suicidal ideation, feelings of hopelessness, self-mutilation by burning herself using cigarettes, extreme anger, loss of appetite, and mood swings. The patient had been hospitalized a total of six times in the last ten years. Since late adolescence she had experienced symptoms of emotional instability, feelings of inferiority, social anxiety, strong ambivalent feelings toward men, episodes of intense anger, dissociative episodes, tendency to be attracted to abusive men, and episodic self-mutilating behavior. She made a serious suicide attempt about five years ago by overdose on a tricyclic antidepressant. She denied drug and alcohol abuse, smoking, and caffeine intake. She was tried on numerous medications in the past, including TCAs, MAOIs, antipsychotics, and mood stabilizers, but there had been no sustained improvement. She was taking trazodone 300 mg prior to her most recent hospitalization. She was sexually abused by her father from age 7 to 13. She was physically abused by all of her three previous husbands. She had been living with her mother until a year ago. Her father had a diagnosis of depression and her grandmother had had a "nervous breakdown." The patient's father died of myocardial infarction when the patient was 22 years old. Her medical history is significant for mitral valve prolapse, supraventricular tachycardia, and gastritis. She had been taking digoxin, verapamil, ranitidine, and metoclopramide.

Axis II Diagnosis: Borderline personality disorder with dependent features

Axis I Diagnosis: Major depression, severe, recurrent

Current Treatment:
1. lithium carbonate 300 mg AM and 600 mg HS
2. bupropion 75 mg TID
3. nortriptyline 25 mg HS
4. trazodone 50 mg HS
5. psychotherapy (intermittently)

Treatment Course: The patient was stabilized in the hospital on the following medications: lithium carbonate 300 mg AM and 600 mg HS, bupropion 75 mg TID, nortriptyline 25 mg HS, and trazodone 50 mg HS. She has been maintained on these medications for the last four years and has been functioning fairly well.

Comments: Most patients with borderline personality disorder tend to become somewhat less emotionally unstable and less dysfunctional as they reach their forties and fifties. They are still prone to depression, especially when faced with interpersonal stresses, and will benefit from a maintenance dose of an antidepressant indefinitely. Since mood instability is one of the common characteristics of borderline personality disorder, a mood stabilizer is also frequently beneficial. I have no reason to believe that the patient has been fairly stable for the last four years because of any unique effects of the current combination of medications. Rather, the improved stability is believed to have resulted from the following factors, with medications possibly playing an important but minor role:

1. Advancing age contributing to maturity and consequent improved stability
2. Relative lack of major interpersonal stresses
3. The patient's adherence to my advice to avoid intimate sexually based relationships (thereby preventing potential stressors)
4. Moderate dependency traits have helped her to be compliant with treatment and have enabled her to accept her mother's support and nurturance
5. Medications

Chapter 7

Histrionic Personality Disorder

DSM-IV diagnostic criteria for histrionic personality disorder are given below.

DSM-IV *CRITERIA AND SYMPTOM CORRELATES*

A pervasive pattern of excessive emotionality and attention seeking, beginning by early childhood and present in a variety of contexts, as indicated by five (or more) of the following:

1. *Is uncomfortable in situations in which he or she is not the center of attention.*
2. *Interaction with others is often characterized by inappropriate sexually seductive or provocative behavior.*
3. *Displays rapidly shifting and shallow expression of emotions.*
4. *Consistently uses physical appearance to draw attention to self.*
5. *Has a style of speech that is excessively impressionistic and lacking in detail.*
6. *Shows self-dramatization, theatricality, and exaggerated expression of emotion.*
7. *Is suggestible, i.e., easily influenced by others or by circumstances.*
8. *Considers relationships to be more intimate than they actually are.*

The symptom correlates that are potentially responsive to currently available medications follow in Table 7.1.

Symptom analysis suggests the possible presence of several treatable symptom clusters.

TABLE 7.1. Symptom Correlates for Histrionic Personality Disorder

***DSM-IV* Criteria**	**Symptom Correlates**
A pervasive pattern of excessive emotionality and attention seeking	increased emotional reactivity, rejection sensitivity, hypomanic features
1. Is uncomfortable in situations in which he or she is not the center of attention	attention-seeking behavior, may suggest a hypomanic feature (could be related to attention deficit disorder symptoms)
2. Interaction with others is often characterized by inappropriate sexually seductive or provocative behavior	suggests a hypomanic feature
3. Displays rapidly shifting and shallow expressions of emotions	emotional liability
4. Consistently uses physical appearance to draw attention to self	may suggest obsessive-compulsive or hypomanic feature
5. Has a style of speech that is excessively impressionistic and lacking in detail	may be variation of pressured speech, suggestive of hypomanic features or attention deficit disorder
6. Shows self-dramatization, theatricality, and exaggerated expression of emotion	excessive emotional reactivity, excessive irritability
7. Is suggestible, i.e., easily influenced by others or circumstances	suggests hypomanic features
8. Considers relationships to be more intimate than they actually are	suggests hypomanic features

Symptom Clusters	Medication Options
Increased emotional sensitivity, rejection sensitivity, obsessive-compulsive features, increased irritability	serotonergic antidepressants, venlafaxine, or nefazodone
Hypomanic features, labile affect, pressured speech, attention deficit disorder	mood stabilizers such as lithium, valproate, or carbamazepine
Attention deficit disorder symptoms	stimulants, bupropion

Depending on the predominant symptoms, either antidepressants or mood stabilizers have a role in the treatment of histrionic personality disorder. If symptoms from the first two clusters are present, first try the patient on an antidepressant medication. If there is still no improvement in symptoms, then discontinue the antidepressant and try a mood stabilizer. If there is partial resolution of symptoms on the antidepressant, but the improvement is suboptimal, a mood stabilizer may be added as an adjunctive medication for better control of symptoms. The reason for initially trying an antidepressant is that often symptoms which present as hypomanic features such as pressured speech and "hyper" behavior are responsive to antidepressants, especially serotonergic medications, perhaps because these symptoms are generated by underlying anxiety, rather than a true manic process. Patients with histrionic personality disorder can present with pseudomanic features which can be easily confused with true mania or hypomania. Table 7.2 lists the differences between true manic features and pseudomania (Joseph, 1997).

Anxiety responds well to serotonergic antidepressants in the low therapeutic dosage range, with no risk of tolerance or dependence. Symptoms of excessive emotional sensitivity, moodiness, lability of affect, and rejection sensitivity are at least partially responsive to treatment using serotonergic antidepressants that offer many advantages including a benign side effect profile, lack of abuse and addiction potential, and improved safety in overdose, among others. Many of the histrionic symptoms could be controlled by seroton-

TABLE 7.2. Characteristics Distinguishing Mania from Pseudomania

	Mania Hypomania	Pseudomania
Severity:	Significant dysfunction in almost all spheres of functioning is common	Dysfunction primarily limited to interpersonal functioning or to one aspect of behavior
Duration:	Behaviors and thoughts persist, lasting days or weeks	Behaviors and thoughts are episodic, lasting hours, but not for days or weeks
Progression:	Behaviors and thoughts tend to worsen if untreated	Behaviors and thoughts return to baseline within hours
Thought Content:	Grandiosity, inflated self-esteem, or extreme hostility are persistent	Grandiosity and increased self-confidence are usually absent; the degree of hostility is less intense, and reactive, and usually directed at close family or co-workers
Rationality:	Irrational thinking is usually present	Irrational thinking is absent
Mood:	Mood may be elevated or irritable, but lability of affect is almost always present	Mood may be irritable, but is not elevated; affect lability is usually absent
Insight:	Usually impaired	Usually preserved
Activity Level:	Reckless, usually unrestrained, repetitive, unremorseful, escalating, and not limited to one type of behavior	Can be excessive, but has a compulsive episodic character, usually limited to one type of behavior, accompanied by guilt, remorse, and distress

Source: Reproduced from S. Joseph, *Symptom-Focused Psychiatric Drug Therapy for Managed Care*, 1997. Binghamton, NY: The Haworth Press.

ergic antidepressants without dysfunctional side effects. Better control of emotions is likely to improve confidence, judgment, impulse control, and frustration tolerance, thereby facilitating the process of emotional maturation which is essential for optimal use of one's other attributes such as intelligence and physical characteristics.

Individuals with histrionic personality disorder are probably at relatively greater risk for reactive depression because of their rather fragile emotional control. They are also prone to develop anxiety disorders and other disorders such as obsessive-compulsive disorders, somatoform disorders, and conversion disorders, where anxiety and suggestibility play a genetic role.

In the case of histrionic personality disorder where symptoms such as pressured speech, labile affect, and hypomanic features approach a variant of cyclothymia, a trial on mood stabilizers is clinically reasonable if SSRIs or bupropion fail.

Coexisting disorders such as adult attention deficit disorder, substance abuse, etc., should be treated using specific agents or techniques, as in any disorder with comorbid conditions.

Many histrionic personality disorder patients will seek treatment for symptoms of anxiety, depression, and moodiness because they are quite vulnerable to developing these symptoms. Fortunately, treatment using serotonergic antidepressants or mood stabilizers will not only improve the presenting complaints, but also modify some of the undesirable personality characteristics.

CLINICAL CASE 31

Case #31

Presenting Symptoms: The patient was a 25-year-old female, with complaints of excessive emotional reactivity, rapid mood swings, attention-seeking behavior, episodic grandiosity, poor frustration tolerance, rejection sensitivity, labile affect,and restlessness. The above symptoms had been present since childhood, according to her parents. The patient was pressured by her husband into seeking psychiatric treatment because of frequent marital conflicts and inconsistent interaction with children. She denied drug and alcohol abuse and smoking. She reported drinking two cups of regular coffee daily. She denied previous psychiatric treatment and a family history of psychiatric disorders. Her medical history is unremarkable.

Axis II Diagnosis: Histrionic personality disorder

Current Treatment: 1. bupropion 150 mg AM and PM
2. risperidone 0.25 mg HS

Treatment Course: The patient reluctantly started sertraline 50 mg AM, which she discontinued after a week because of sexual dysfunction. Several months later, the medication was started again under pressure from her husband and family members. She took the medication for a month and stopped again on her own. Sertraline was restarted about six months later, and increased to 100 mg AM. The medication was discontinued because of lack of response. After trials on other SSRIs, the patient was placed on bupropion 75 mg BID, eventually increased to 150 mg BID and risperidone 0.25 mg HS. Risperidone at a very low dose was added to control episodic hostility. Her symptoms responded satisfactorily on the current combinations of medications.

Comments: Histrionic personality disorder can present with symptoms suggestive of various disorders, such as anxiety disorders, hypomania, depression, obsessive-compulsive disorder, attention deficit disorder, and mild forms of rapid-cycling bipolar disorder. However, the patient does not meet the full criteria for the disorders listed above. For example, the mood swings seen in histrionic personality disorder do not reach the amplitudes often seen in bipolar disorder. As emphasized throughout this book, the presence of symptoms merits treatment. In this particular patient, emotional instability and sensitivity were the predominant symptoms that responded to bupropion, but not to SSRIs. If hypomanic symptoms are predominant, a mood stabilizer might be tried. In many cases with personality disorders, apparent hypomanic symptoms respond well to antidepressants, particularly to SSRIs. Antipsychotic medication is rarely necessary for treatment of histrionic personality disorder. In general, antidepressants are sufficient with the use of mood stabilizers in select patients. Since SSRI antidepressants are safe and less complicated medications, they are given a full trial prior to trying or adding mood stabilizers. It is tempting for clinicians to overdiagnose histrionic personality disorder due to patients' histrionic presentation. Often, the diagnosis of bipolar disorder or cyclothymia is erroneously made and patients are started on mood stabilizers. However, it is possible that histrionic personality disorder can present with other low-level symptoms, some of which may need independent treatment using various medications.

If the patient's mood swings do not respond to SSRIs or other antidepressants, it is reasonable to try the patient on a mood stabilizer such as lithium, valproic acid, carbamazepine, gabapentin, or lamotrigine.

Psychoanalysis or psychoanalytically oriented psychotherapy is considered the therapy of choice for histrionic personality disorder. In my view, psychotherapy, initiated while the patient is stabilized on medication, provides the best results in terms of rapid resolution of symptoms. The medication may be slowly tapered off after one to two years. However, some patients experience a relapse of symptoms in which case medication may need to be reinstituted for a longer period of time.

Chapter 8

Narcissistic Personality Disorder

The *DSM-IV* criteria for narcissistic personality are below.

DSM-IV *CRITERIA AND SYMPTOM CORRELATES*

A pervasive pattern of grandiosity (in fantasy or behavior), need for admiration, and lack of empathy, beginning by early adulthood and present in a variety of contexts, as indicated by five (or more) of the following:

1. *Has a grandiose sense of self-importance (e.g., exaggerates achievements and talents, expects to be recognized as superior without commensurate achievements).*
2. *Is preoccupied with fantasies of unlimited success, power, brilliance, beauty, or ideal love.*
3. *Believes that he or she is "special" and unique and can only be understood by, or should associate with, other special or high-status people (or institutions).*
4. *Requires excessive admiration.*
5. *Has a sense of entitlement, i.e., unreasonable expectations of especially favorable treatment or automatic compliance with his or her expectations.*
6. *Is interpersonally exploitative, i.e., takes advantage of others to achieve his or her ends.*
7. *Lacks empathy, i.e., is unwilling to recognize or identify with the feelings and needs of others.*

---

8. Is often envious of others or believes that others are envious of him or her.
9. Shows arrogant, haughty behaviors or attitudes.

The symptom correlates that are potentially treatable with currently available medications are listed in Table 8.1.

An analysis of the symptom correlates points to predominantly hypomanic characteristics as well as the possibility of mild paranoia. The major medication classes likely to improve these symptoms are:

Symptom Clusters	Possible Medication Options
Hypomanic (predominant)	mood stabilizers and/or antipsychotics
Mild paranoia/hostility (infrequent)	low dose of antipsychotics (risperidone, olanzapine, or sertindole preferred)

Some of the dysfunctional features of narcissistic personality disorder can possibly be improved on mood stabilizers such as lithium, valproate, carbamazepine, gabapentin, or lamotrigine. Since risperidone presents a better side effect profile including decreased extrapyramidal reactions, and possibly decreased incidence of tardive dyskinesia, it is an excellent option as a first-line adjunctive antipsychotic medication—either along with a mood stabilizer or as a single agent. At very low doses such as 0.25 to 0.5 mg, or 1 mg of risperidone, the acute side effects are likely to be minimal and the medication is well tolerated. Surprisingly, patients respond nicely to what may appear to be a subtherapeutic dose of 0.25 to 0.5 mg of risperidone daily. Since the side effects in long-term use of risperidone are not yet known, the author is unable to make definitive comments on this topic. However, since the dosage is very low and since risperidone is thought to have a low incidence of typical long-term neuroleptic side effects usually associated with traditional antipsychotics, risperidone at a dosage of 0.25 to 0.5 mg daily is likely to have only minimal, if any, serious neuroleptic side effects. Antipsychotics can be used for short-term control of hypomania and mania. In fact, antipsychotics are preferred (along with concurrent use of benzodiazepines) for acute control of a floridly manic patient. Antipsychotics are effective for the management of

TABLE 8.1. Symptom Correlates for Narcissistic Personality Disorder

	***DSM-IV* Criteria**	**Possible Symptom Correlates**
1.	Has a grandiose sense of self-importance (e.g., exaggerates achievements and talents, expects to be recognized as superior without commensurate achievements)	hypomanic symptoms
2.	Is preoccupied with fantasies of unlimited success, power, brilliance, beauty, or ideal love	hypomanic symptoms
3.	Believes that he or she is "special" and unique and can be only understood by, or should associate with, other special or high-status people (or institutions)	hypomanic symptoms
4.	Requires excessive admiration	hypomanic symptoms
5.	Has a sense of entitlement, i.e., unreasonable expectations of especially favorable treatment or automatic compliance with his or her expectations	hypomanic symptoms
6.	Is interpersonally exploitative, i.e., takes advantage of others to achieve his or her own ends	*antisocial features
7.	Lacks empathy–is unwilling to recognize or identify with the feelings and needs of others	antisocial features
8.	Is often envious of others or believes that others are envious of him or her	mild paranoia/hostility
9.	Shows arrogant, haughty behaviors or attitudes	hypomania/hostility

Note: *Effective medication treatment not currently available.

mania and for prophylaxis. The primary reason that antipsychotics should not be used for long-term prophylaxis of mania is not because they are not effective, but because they have potentially disabling side effects (e.g., tardive dyskinesia) in long-term use. Thus, if an antipsychotic can be developed which has a low risk of acute and long-term side effects, theoretically that antipsychotic could be used for the treatment of acute mania, hypomania, and for prophylaxis. Risperidone, olanzapine, and sertindole tend to come fairly close to the above ideal, among the antipsychotics available presently. Given the possibility that some narcissistic personalities have mild paranoid tendencies and hostility, a trial of a low dose of risperidone, olanzapine, or sertindole is potentially beneficial to the patient. Obviously, if an antipsychotic at low doses is to be tried, the first choice should be risperidone, olanzapine, or sertindole because of reasons already described.

Mood stabilizers alone may be sufficient to give some therapeutic benefits to individuals with narcissistic personality disorder, in which case they are the preferred and primary medications. Important pharmacologic and clinical profiles of mood stabilizers are described in the author's book *Symptom-Focused Psychiatric Drug Therapy for Managed Care*, 1997.

Individuals with narcissistic personality disorder are at high risk for developing depression, primarily due to interpersonal conflicts and other frustrations likely to arise when their expectation of special consideration, regard, and admiration are not fulfilled. They seem particularly vulnerable to dysphoric irritability and dysphoric hypomania, both of which may respond to either antidepressants, mood stabilizers, or a combination of these medications. Among antidepressants SSRIs are preferred due to their improved side effect profile. If the dysphoria or hypomania has an angry or irritable quality, short-term use of a low dose of risperidone, olanzapine, sertindole, or another high-potency antipsychotic might help. Refer to Chapter 15 for a detailed discussion of the clnical profiles of risperidone, olanzapine, and sertindole.

Narcissistic personality disorders typically present to clinical attention due to Axis I symptoms such as depression or anxiety, as is true of all personality disorders. Identification of the dysfunctional personality characteristics often requires collateral information from a significant other who is often affected by the patient's narcissistic attitudes and behavior. Both Axis I and Axis II symptoms must be identified and specifically treated for optimal and lasting improvement.

CLINICAL CASES 32 to 35

Case #32

Presenting Symptoms: The patient was a 30-year-old male, with symptoms consisting of conflicts with his wife, exploitative behavior, excessive emotional sensitivity, mild hypomania, mild mood swings, procrastination, perfectionistic tendencies, frequent lying to conceal his exploits, anxiety, inflated self-importance, distractibility, depressed mood, difficulty focusing, excessive self-centeredness, and indifference to others' feelings. Most of the symptoms had been present for many years. Psychiatric evaluation and treatment were initiated at the urging of his wife who provided a good part of the history. He denied drug and alcohol abuse, smoking, and caffeine intake. He had taken fluoxetine 20 mg off and on in the past. His father had a history of bipolar disorder (manic), and his mother had a history of obsessive-compulsive disorder and hypomanic episodes. (The author had the privilege of treating both parents.)

Axis II Diagnosis: Narcissistic personality disorder with obsessive-compulsive features

Axis I Diagnosis: Mild attention deficit disorder (ADD)

Current Treatment:
1. lithium (Eskalith CR) 450 mg HS
2. fluvoxamine 100 mg HS
3. risperidone 0.25 mg (1/4th of a 1 mg pill) HS
4. methylphenidate 5 mg BID
5. referral for psychotherapy

Treatment Course: The patient was given Eskalith CR 225 mg BID, risperidone 0.5 mg HS, and fluvoxamine 50 mg HS at the first visit. Encouraged by some improvement, the author increased fluvoxamine to 100 mg at the second visit and to 150 mg HS at the third office visit. Although obsessive-compulsive symptoms improved to the patient's satisfaction with fluvoxamine 150 mg HS, the dose was eventually decreased to 100 mg HS at the patient's request because of increasing sexual dysfunction, which was troubling to the patient. Since the patient continued to complain of distractibility, restlessness, and difficulty in focusing, methylphenidate 5 mg AM and PM was added with good results. The dose of risperidone was recently decreased to 0.25 mg, and could be discontinued at the next visit in three months. The lithium level was at 0.4 mEq/L. All presenting symptoms have subsided for the most part on the current medications to the extent that he has been getting along well with his wife and his co-workers. The patient had previously believed that he was born with his "attitudes and temperament" and that they were not amenable to change. He is surprised at his newly found maturity and responsible behavior.

Comments: Most patients with personality disorders hesitantly seek psychiatric evaluation and treatment upon the insistence of a family member, employer, or the court system. Personality disorders frequently lead to interpersonal conflicts causing secondary depression, anxiety, insomnia, etc. When the patients present to the clinician's office primarily to appease the referral source, they are typically not very forthcoming with history of their present illness. Because of this problem, collateral information from a family member, employer, the court system or other referral source is extremely useful in arriving at the correct diagnosis. Besides, personality disorders frequently manifest in behaviors in an interpersonal or social context and these behavior patterns are usually better observed by others. The patients themselves might be oblivious to these behavior tendencies unless they are quite perceptive, unlike an Axis I condition such as anxiety or depressive disorders, where the patients' intense subjective distress is generally obvious and something they feel.

Among personality disorders, narcissistic, antisocial, schizoid, and paranoid personality disorders are, in the author's experience, the most difficult to engage in treatment. The devaluation of the treatment, the clinician, and others by the narcissistic patient is more sustained than by the borderline patient's devaluation (which is changeable). However, if a narcissistic patient can be persuaded to accept treatment, various medications can be beneficial. A mood stabilizer and/or a low dose of an antipsychotic can improve the chronic hypomania that is common in narcissistic patients.

This particular patient's symptoms can be grouped into the following clusters. Medications were chosen to address each symptom group. Specific medication choices under each medication group can vary among practitioners.

Symptom Group	Medication Group	Specific Medication
hypomanic	mood stabilizer and/or antipsychotic	lithium risperidone
obsessive-compulsive	antiobsessional	fluvoxamine
mild depressive	antidepressant	fluvoxamine
ADD	stimulant	methylphenidate

Since most personality disorders present symptoms overlapping with other disorders (as is also true of Axis I disorders), a variety of medications from different classes are usually necessary. The specific dosage of medications from different classes determines the relative "weights" and thereby provides the unique balance. This is where the art of medical practice takes over. However, I believe that this is an art that can be learned.

Case #33

Presenting Symptoms: The patient was a 40-year-old male, whose symptoms consisted of depressed mood, anxiety, irritability, grandiosity, impatience, mild suspiciousness, excessive anger, arrogance, insomnia, feelings of hopelessness, compulsive tendencies, excessive emotional sensitivity, sense of entitlement, and alcohol dependence. All of the symptoms except depressive symptoms had been present since early adulthood. He had been drinking eight to ten beers daily for several years. He smoked marijuana (five "joints") daily. The depressive symptoms were precipitated by a business failure. The patient sought psychiatric services after his wife separated and threatened divorce. The psychiatric history was significant for a 14-day inpatient treatment for substance abuse ten years ago. He denied smoking cigarettes and caffeine intake. The patient was recently seen by another psychiatrist who refused to treat him because the psychiatrist and the patient had a "personality conflict," and the psychiatrist became angry and told the patient that he was "untreatable," as reported by the patient. He denied any family history of psychiatric problems, and also denied any active medical problems.

Axis II Diagnosis: Narcissistic personality disorder with mild paranoid and obsessive-compulsive features

Axis I Diagnosis: Major depression, moderate, single episode
Alcohol dependence
Cannabis dependence

Current Treatment:
1. paroxetine 20 mg AM
2. risperidone 0.5 mg HS
3. trazodone 50 mg HS
4. naltrexone 50 mg PM
5. referral to Alcoholics Anonymous and to a psychotherapist

Treatment Course: The patient was started on all of the following medications at the first office visit.

1. chlordiazepoxide 10 mg–take 80 mg the first night and decrease by 20 mg daily until completed (in four days)
2. thiamine 100 mg QD for seven days
3. multivitamin one tablet QD for 30 days
4. paroxetine 20 mg AM
5. risperidone 0.5 mg HS
6. trazodone 25 mg HS
7. naltrexone 50 mg PM

When the patient was seen one week later, he reported marked improvement. Trazodone was increased to 50 mg HS to treat insomnia. He was seen two weeks later. Since mild depressive symptoms and anxiety persisted, paroxetine was increased to 30 mg AM. The patient had satisfactory resolution of symptoms, including personality disorder symptoms, on the current combination of medications, which are expected to be maintained for six months to one year.

Comments: Patients with narcissistic personality disorder typically come to clinical attention either due to external pressure or due to distressing Axis I symptoms such as depression, anxiety, insomnia, substance abuse, suicidality, etc. They rarely, if ever, come to the clinician only to report symptoms such as grandiosity, paranoia, sense of entitlement, hostility, or arrogance. However, when they present to the clinician with Axis I symptoms, there is the opportunity to treat both Axis I and Axis II symptoms. The following medications probably were effective in improving the Axis II symptoms in this patient.

Axis II Symptoms	Medication
Grandiosity, paranoia, entitlement	risperidone
Arrogance, hostility, impatience	paroxetine

The comment which suggested that his personality disorder symptoms had improved was from his wife of 18 years who, after one month of starting this treatment, told him, "I hadn't known that you could be such a likeable man."

Case #34

Presenting Symptoms: The patient was a 40-year-old male, with symptoms consisting of depressed mood, anhedonia, suicidal ideation, feelings of hopelessness, crying episodes, increased anxiety, anger attacks, and a history of hypomanic episodes. The depression was precipitated by a recent marital separation. His premorbid personality pattern is characterized by grandiosity, arrogant attitudes, feelings of superiority, lack of empathy, mild paranoia, tendency to be exploitive in interpersonal relationships, labile affect, and excessive preoccupation with physical appearance. He denied drug and alcohol abuse, and smoking. He reported drinking two cups of coffee daily. He also denied a family history of psychiatric disorders.

Axis II Diagnosis: Narcissistic personality disorder with histrionic features

Axis I Diagnosis: Bipolar disorder, depressed

Current Treatment:
1. lithium (Eskalith CR) 225 mg AM and 450 mg HS
2. risperidone 0.5 mg HS

3. nefazodone 150 mg BID
4. psychotherapy

Treatment Course: The patient was hospitalized for five days and discharged on the medications listed above. Lithium level was 0.5 mEq/L. Depression and most of the personality disorder symptoms improved significantly on these medications. Thyroid profile has been within the normal range.

Comments: Information obtained from the patient's wife indicated that it was the patient's chronically self-centered and arrogant attitudes and behaviors that were primarily responsible for ongoing marital conflicts which ultimately led to the marital separation that precipitated the depression. As is true with regard to almost all cases presented in this book, Axis II disorders directly or indirectly precipitate Axis I disorders that bring the patient to clinical attention. However, for optimal outcome, it is important to treat both the acute Axis I and the chronic Axis II symptoms. If the Axis II symptoms are not addressed, the patient is likely to continue to have interpersonal or intrapersonal problems, which will predispose to the emergence of Axis I symptoms sooner or later.

Case #35

Presenting Symptoms: The patient was a 36-year-old male, whose symptoms consisted of depressed mood, anger outbursts, racing thoughts, violence toward his wife and stepson, grandiosity, impatience, manipulative behavior, impulsivity, legal problems (a history of three arrests), irritability, suspiciousness, ideas of reference, distrust of others, insomnia, and paranoid ideation. The patient sought treatment after his wife threatened him with divorce if he did not receive psychiatric treatment. He had been smoking marijuana, and using cocaine episodically. He smoked one pack of cigarettes per day and drank three cups of coffee daily. The patient's wife described him as selfish, controlling, suspicious, and dishonest for the ten years that they had been married. His own reports suggest that at least some of the above characteristics had been present for 15 to 20 years. He denied alcohol abuse. Both of the patient's parents had suffered from alcoholism, his mother had been diagnosed with severe depression and had attempted suicide once, and his sister was schizophrenic.

Axis II Diagnosis:	Narcissistic personality disorder with paranoid and antisocial features
Axis I Diagnosis:	Dysthymia Consider bipolar II
Current Treatment:	1. divalproex sodium 250 mg AM and 500 mg HS 2. paroxetine 30 mg AM 3. risperidone 1.5 mg HS 4. clonazepam 0.5 mg HS 5. psychotherapy

Treatment Course: The patient was given fluoxetine up to 40 mg with no significant improvement. He was switched to paroxetine 20 mg and eventually increased to 30 mg. Divalproex sodium, risperidone, and clonazepam were sequentially added to control discrete symptom groups. His symptoms are well-controlled on the current medications and dosages.

Comments: The patients' symptoms can be classified into several symptom groups based on medication responsiveness as follows:

Symptom Group	Medication Class	Specific Medication
Hypomania, grandiosity, racing thoughts, violent behavior	mood stabilizer	divalproex sodium
Depressed mood, irritability	antidepressant	paroxetine
Suspiciousness, ideas of reference, impulsivity, distrust, paranoia	antipsychotic	risperidone
Insomnia	hypnotic benzodiazepine	clonazepam

Since most personality disorders present with a variety of symptoms that need medications from different classes, a combination of medications is typically necessary for the best outcome. Even most of the complicated personality disorders (as this one) are treatable with sufficient and sustained external pressure and the right balance of medications along with psychotherapy. Symptom analysis and symptom-focused treatment are the keys to achieving a successful outcome.

Chapter 9

Avoidant Personality Disorder

The diagnostic criteria of avoidant personality disorder according to *DSM-IV* are given below.

DSM-IV *CRITERIA AND SYMPTOM CORRELATES*

A pervasive pattern of social inhibition, feelings of inadequacy, and hypersensitivity to negative evaluation, beginning in early adulthood and present in a variety of contexts, as indicated by four (or more) of the following:

1. *Avoids occupational activities that involve significant interpersonal contact, because of fears of criticism, disapproval, or rejection.*
2. *Is unwilling to get involved with people unless certain of being liked.*
3. *Shows restraint within intimate relationships because of the fear of being shamed or ridiculed.*
4. *Is preoccupied with being criticized or rejected in social situations.*
5. *Is inhibited in new interpersonal situations because of feelings of inadequacy.*
6. *Views self as socially inept, personally unappealing, or inferior to others.*
7. *Is unusually reluctant to take personal risks or to engage in any new activities because they may prove embarrassing.*

The symptom correlates that are possibly responsive to currently available medications follow in Table 9.1.

An analysis of the symptom correlates indicates that avoidant personality disorder is primarily characterized by social phobia, social anxiety, performance anxiety, agoraphobia and rejection sensitivity. These patients are at high risk for developing Axis I disorders, such as generalized anxiety disorder, panic disorder with agoraphobia, and depression, which represent the most frequent presenting complaints. These symptoms respond to MAOIs such as phenelzine or tranylcypromine, SSRIs, venlafaxine, and nefazodone; or benzodiaze-

TABLE 9.1. Symptom Correlates for Avoidant Personality Disorder

***DSM-IV* Criteria**	**Symptom Correlates**
A pervasive pattern of social inhibition, feelings of inadequacy, and hypersensitivity to negative evaluation, beginning in early adulthood and present in a variety of contexts	social phobia, social anxiety, performance anxiety, excessive emotional sensitivity
1. Avoids occupational activities that involve significant interpersonal contact, because of fears of criticism, disapproval, or rejection	rejection sensitivity
2. Is unwilling to get involved with people unless certain of being liked	social anxiety
3. Shows restraint within intimate relationships because of the fear of being shamed or ridiculed	anxiety
4. Is preoccupied with being criticized or rejected in social situations	social phobia
5. Is inhibited in new situations because of feelings of inadequacy	social anxiety
6. Views self as socially inept, personally unappealing, or inferior to others	poor self-esteem, feelings of inadequacy
7. Is unusually reluctant to take personal risks or to engage in any new activities because they may prove embarrassing	performance anxiety

pines such as alprazolam and clonazepam; and beta-blockers, or combinations of the above medications. Possible treatable symptom clusters and medication options are listed in Table 9.2.

If one agent alone is only partially effective, other medications can be sequentially added for increased effectiveness. MAOIs are effective for the treatment of the symptom clusters related to avoidant personality disorder. The anticholinergic side effects, dietary restrictions, and potentially dangerous medication interactions associated with MAOIs have discouraged their routine use, even for the treatment of symptoms that are known to respond well to them. SSRIs have the significant advantage of a benign side effect profile, lack of dietary restrictions, and compatibility with most other medications. Moreover, SSRIs seem to be as effective as MAOIs in controlling all of the social anxiety symptoms associated with avoidant personality disorder. The choices among these medications include fluoxetine, sertraline, paroxetine, venlafaxine, fluvoxamine, and nefazodone. An option among TCAs is clomipramine, which has excellent antianxiety and antiphobic effects. One approach is to keep patients on an SSRI or an MAOI as a primary agent and to add a benzodiazepine such as alprazolam or clonazepam, or to add a beta-blocker or a combination of a benzodiazepine and a beta-blocker to the primary agent on a PRN basis, for example, on occasions such as a social function or a dating engagement when the acutely high anxi-

TABLE 9.2. Symptom-Based Medication Guide for Avoidant Personality Disorder

Symptom Clusters	Medication Options
Social anxiety, social phobia, rejection sensitivity, performance anxiety, anticipatory anxiety, excessive emotional sensitivity	SSRIs, venlafaxine, nefazodone, MAOIs, benzodiazepines, (alprazolam, clonazepam, etc.), beta-blockers

Combinations:

1. SSRI and benzodiazepine
2. SSRI, benzodiazepine, and beta-blocker
3. benzodiazepine and beta-blocker
4. SSRI and beta-blocker
5. MAOI and benzodiazepine
6. MAOI, benzodiazepine, and beta-blocker
7. MAOI and beta-blocker

ety is likely to interfere with optimal functioning. Although MAOIs and SSRIs have prophylaxis against anxiety symptoms, they do not act acutely and are not effective for acute prophylactic effects for dealing with occasions when breakthrough anxiety is likely. Benzodiazepines and beta-blockers are much more effective, and are excellent for sporadic use. They are the medications of choice for treating phobia if the phobic stimulus is present only infrequently; however, if the phobic stimulus has to be confronted fairly frequently, it is more efficient to treat the patient using a primary medication such as an MAOI or an SSRI. Since the social phobia present in Avoidant Personality Disorder is more of a pervasive or generalized type, long-term treatment on a primary medication is necessary for maximum effectiveness. Occasional use of benzodiazepines and beta-blockers adjunctively is still beneficial in these patients.

Behavioral-cognitive therapy using social skills training, relaxation training, and graded desensitization training, etc., are some of the psychotherapeutic approaches that should help most individuals with avoidant personality disorder. Clinical experience overwhelmingly shows that once the patient's symptoms are fairly controlled on medication, he or she is able to benefit more from the psychotherapeutic approach, rather than the other way around.

If avoidant characteristics are extreme, the clinician should carefully search for underlying paranoia, psychotically based fear, and psychotic withdrawal. In the author's experience, severe avoidant symptoms were frequently found to have a psychotic component that responded well to the addition of an antipsychotic, or to an antipsychotic alone. Although the clinician should rule out underlying psychosis in all patients as a matter of routine clinical assessment, it is particularly important to suspect underlying psychosis in avoidant personalities simply because prodromal, residual, and atypical psychoses can present with avoidant symptoms.

CLINICAL CASE 36

Case #36

Presenting Symptoms: The patient was a 16-year-old female, whose symptoms consisted of avoidance of social relationships, excessive self-consciousness, feelings of inferiority, reluctance to go to school because of fear of being ridiculed or criticized, social anxiety, depressed mood, recent anxiety attacks, initial insomnia, decreased appetite, and excessive worrying. The patient's mother described the patient as being habitually shy, but the avoidance behavior had gradually been getting worse since age 13. She denied drug and alcohol abuse, smoking, and caffeine intake. The patient's two aunts suffered from "depression and anxiety." She denied a history of medical problems, except for frequent heartburn.

Axis II Diagnosis: Avoidant personality disorder

Axis I Diagnosis: Panic disorder with agoraphobia
Consider social phobia, generalized type

Current Treatment:
1. paroxetine 20 mg AM
2. imipramine 25 mg HS
3. alprazolam 0.25 mg PRN (1-2 times a week)
4. ranitidine 150 mg HS
5. referral for psychotherapy

Treatment Course: Several symptom groups were identified as follows:

Symptom Group	Medication Group	Specific Medication
Avoidant symptoms	antidepressant	paroxetine
Anxiety attacks	antidepressant benzodiazepine	paroxetine
Depressive symptoms	antidepressant	paroxetine
Insomnia	hypnotic	(imipramine)
Loss of appetite	TCA	imipramine
Dyspepsia	H2 blocker	ranitidine

At the first office visit, the patient was started on paroxetine 10 mg AM, imipramine 10 mg HS, and ranitidine 150 mg BID. Note that paroxetine and imipramine were at very low doses. At the next office visit two weeks later, she reported moderate improvement with no side effects. The dose of paroxetine was increased to 20 mg

AM, and ranitidine was decreased to 150 mg HS. Since the patient continued to complain of insomnia and anorexia, the dose of imipramine was increased to 25 mg HS during a subsequent visit, with good results. Alprazolam 0.25 mg was prescribed for PRN use. The patient has been taking alprazolam at an average frequency of one to two per week. Her Axis I as well as Axis II symptoms subsided to the point that she has become asymptomatic.

Comments: There is considerable overlap between symptoms of avoidant personality disorder and Axis I conditions such as social phobia and agoraphobia. It is at times difficult to distinguish between symptoms of avoidant personality disorder and social phobia. Either of these diagnoses could be reasonable in a particular case. In these situations the author tends to favor the diagnosis of social phobia on Axis I because of an open bias toward diagnosis of an Axis I disorder whenever possible.

Since the choice of treatment is dictated by the specific symptom configuration, according to the symptom-focused treatment approach, the formal diagnosis is not as important immediately as is the identification of all of the distressing symptoms.

In general, phobic, anxiety, and avoidant symptoms respond well to antidepressants along with use of a low dose of one of the potent benzodiazepines on a PRN schedule. Prior to the advent of SSRIs, two of the antidepressants that were used in the treatment of social phobia were imipramine and phenelzine. The author's choice of imipramine to treat insomnia and anorexia was influenced by its independent beneficial effects on phobic and avoidance symptoms.

It should be emphasized that avoidant and social phobic symptoms appearing in adolescence or in early adulthood could be prodromal symptoms of schizophrenia; hence, it is important to rule out this diagnosis and to continue to monitor the patient for possible emergence of schizophrenia because the treatment is substantially different. If social phobia and avoidance are severe, the presence of underlying paranoia or psychotic processes should be strongly suspected and treatment changed accordingly.

Chapter 10

Dependent Personality Disorder

The diagnostic criteria for diagnosis of dependent personality disorder according to *DSM-IV* are as follows.

DSM-IV *CRITERIA AND SYMPTOM CORRELATES*

A pervasive and excessive need to be taken care of that leads to submissive and clinging behavior and fears of separation, beginning in early adulthood and present in a variety of contexts, as indicated by five (or more) of the following:

1. *Has difficulty making everyday decisions without an excessive amount of advice and reassurance from others.*
2. *Needs others to assume responsibility for most major areas of his or her life.*
3. *Has difficulty expressing disagreement with others because of fear of loss of support or approval. (Note: Do not include realistic fears of retribution.)*
4. *Has difficulty initiating projects or doing things on his or her own (because of a lack of self-confidence in judgement or abilities rather than a lack of motivation or energy).*
5. *Goes to excessive lengths to obtain nurturance and support from others, to the point of volunteering to do things that are unpleasant.*
6. *Feels uncomfortable or helpless when alone because of exaggerated fears of being unable to care for himself or herself.*

---

7. *Urgently seeks another relationship as a source of care and support when a close relationship ends.*
8. *Is unrealistically preoccupied with fears of being left to take care of himself or herself.*

The symptom correlates that are potentially responsive to medication treatment are listed in Table 10.1.

Since all of the behavior patterns suggest the presence of symptoms such as anxiety and depression, any attempts at medication treatment should be directed to these symptoms. The first-line medications for depression and anxiety in modern psychiatric practice are the serotonergic antidepressants, venlafaxine, mirtazapine, and nefazodone because of their favorable side effect profiles and their effectiveness in the treatment of anxiety. However, all antidepressants including MAOIs, trazodone, TCAs and bupropion, should be effective. In addition to antidepressant treatment, patients with Dependent Personality Disorder may benefit from adjunctive treatment using antianxiety medications, either on a standing basis or, preferably, on a PRN schedule.

Patients with dependent personality disorder almost always present with Axis I symptoms such as depression and anxiety. Excessive dependency makes them quite vulnerable to reacting with depression and/or anxiety in the face of interpersonal separation, threats of separation, or interpersonal conflicts. Their dependency also generates subconscious hostility toward the individual on whom they are dependent. There seems to be a low level of dysthymia inherent in patients with dependent traits; therefore, they have the

TABLE 10.1. Symptom Correlates for Dependent Personality Disorder

DSM-IV **Criteria**	**Symptom Correlates**
A pervasive and excessive need to be taken care of that leads to submissive and clinging behavior and fears of separation, beginning in early adulthood and present in a variety of contexts	anxiety, depression

potential to benefit from antidepressants on a fairly long-term schedule–even if major depressive symptoms are not evident. Psychotherapy is likely to be more effective if the patient is pretreated with an antidepressant medication.

Psychotherapeutic approaches have a particularly important role in the treatment of patients with dependent personality disorder. Their dependency makes them especially good candidates for psychotherapy. The goal of successful therapy is that of ameliorating the dysfunctional and excessive dependency characteristics.

The combination of medications and psychotherapy tends to have a synergistic effect for nearly all symptoms, with medication providing fairly rapid symptom relief, and psychotherapy providing conflict resolution, reassurance, psychological support, insight, acceptance, understanding, and psychosocial coping skills, which are important goals in a comprehensive treatment approach. If dependency reaches regressive proportions, the presence of underlying psychosis, especially characterized by negative symptoms, must be carefully explored.

CLINICAL CASES 37 to 40

Case #37

Presenting Symptoms: The patient was a 42-year-old female, with symptoms consisting of depressed mood, crying episodes, panic attacks, increased anxiety, and feelings of hopelessness precipitated by a divorce about one year ago. The patient was accompanied to the office by her mother. Further history obtained from the patient and her mother indicated that since late adolescence the patient had a tendency to be excessively dependent on her parents or her husband for making decisions related to her personal and vocational choices. She also had excessive fear of rejection by others, a clinging neediness, and a recurrent fear of being abandoned by others. The patient denied drug and alcohol abuse, and caffeine intake. She reported smoking two packs of cigarettes per day. She had had several episodes of depression about five years ago and was then treated with nortriptyline. Fluoxetine made her "hyper." The patient's mother had a diagnosis of depression, which was being treated with paroxetine. The patient's medical history is significant for chronic back pain.

Axis II Diagnosis: Dependent personality disorder

Axis I Diagnosis: Major depression, moderate, recurrent
Panic disorder without agoraphobia

Current Treatment: 1. paroxetine 30 mg AM and 15 mg noon
2. alprazolam 0.5 mg TID PRN
3. referral for psychotherapy

Treatment Course: The patient was placed on paroxetine 20 mg AM and alprazolam 0.5 mg po BID-TID PRN for severe anxiety at the first office visit. Paroxetine was gradually increased to the current dose of 45 mg daily to achieve the best response. The patient takes alprazolam 0.5 mg four to five times a week on the average. The patient reported that depressive and anxiety symptoms as well as most of the symptoms indicative of dependent personality disorder improved after starting the antidepressant.

Comments: As is true with all personality disorders, patients typically present with acute symptoms suggestive of Axis I disorders. Nonspecific symptoms such as depressed mood, anxiety, and insomnia constitute the great majority of presenting symptoms. The diagnosis of a personality disorder is based on longitudinal historical information that reveals chronic patterns of behavior, attitudes, and feelings. Collateral information from close family members is usually very helpful in making an accurate diagnosis. Excessive dependency in an adult leads to feelings of insecurity, inadequacy, helplessness, and worthlessness, and readily predisposes the individual to clinical depression and anxiety disorders. Any interpersonal conflict or separation can be a precipitant.

Treatment using an antidepressant and PRN use of high-potency benzodiazepines such as alprazolam, clonazepam, and lorazepam is very effective in partially ameliorating dependency symptoms. The preferred antidepressants for use with patients who have dependent personality disorder, in my clinical experience, tend to be SSRIs, which seem to more effectively enhance self-confidence and improve social anxiety as well as to more effectively decrease excessive interpersonal sensitivity and neediness, when compared to TCAs. Adjunctive use of benzodiazepines on a PRN basis provides excellent coverage for breakthrough anxiety, giving patients a sense of control over their difficulties, without the risk of dependence, whereas treatment using antidepressants provides secondary and tertiary prevention.

Case #38

Presenting Symptoms: The patient was a 34-year-old female, whose symptoms consisted of depressed mood, feelings of hopelessness, helplessness, and worthlessness, a history of three suicide attempts, crying episodes, irritability, poor self- confidence, suicidal ideation, difficulty being assertive, excessive reliance on her boyfriend and/or family members, and excessive fear of abandonment and rejection. These symptoms worsened after a recent breakup with her boyfriend. The patient's dependency traits had been present since her early twenties. She was hospitalized twice previously, both precipitated by a breakup of a heterosexual relationship. She denied drug and alcohol abuse, smoking, and caffeine intake. She was taking doxepin 100 mg HS and alprazolam 0.25 mg TID PRN when seen at my office. Her brother abused her sexually at age nine. She denied a family history of psychiatric disorders. The patient also denied major medical problems.

Axis II Diagnosis: Dependent personality disorder

Axis I Diagnosis: Major depression, severe, recurrent
dysthymia

Current Treatment:
1. venlafaxine 150 mg AM and 100 mg PM
2. bupropion 100 mg AM
3. trazodone 50 mg HS PRN for insomnia
4. psychotherapy

Treatment Course: Doxepin was discontinued because of excessive weight gain. While being switched to venlafaxine, the patient had to be hospitalized after she became severely depressed, again precipitated by a breakup with her boyfriend. She was discharged after a four-day hospitalization during which the dose of venlafaxine was increased to 75 mg TID. The dosing schedule was later changed to a more convenient schedule of 150 mg AM and 100 mg

PM. Bupropion 100 mg AM was added for treatment of anergia. Trazodone 50 mg HS is taken occasionally for insomnia. The patient's Axis I depressive symptoms resolved rapidly. Axis II dependency symptoms have shown moderate and sustained improvement so far. Psychotherapy has been a major factor in her recovery.

Comments: The author believes that symptoms of dependent personality disorder will show improvement if treated with antidepressant medication in the context of cognitive-behavioral oriented psychotherapy. In actual practice experience, virtually all patients with dependent personality disorder present with symptoms of depression and/or anxiety. Extreme dependency that is regressive and dysfunctional in nature could suggest an underlying psychotic process and might need adjunctive treatment using antipsychotics. Dependent traits are very common and at moderate levels may even be desirable for maintenance of long-term relationships. The problem arises when dependency traits are excessive to the point that the person feels helpless and insecure by him or herself. Dependent individuals also risk being easy targets of abuse and exploitation by the dominant partner.

Case #39

Presenting Symptoms: The patient was a 48-year-old female, with symptoms consisting of depressed mood, suicidal ideation with intent and plan to shoot herself, frequent crying, severe insomnia, loss of appetite, feelings of hopelessness and helplessness, anhedonia, and anxiety. These symptoms were precipitated by a recent divorce. Her premorbid personality pattern is characterized by symptoms such as chronic feelings of helplessness and worthlessness, subservient attitudes and behavior, excessive dependence on a male partner, fear of being abandoned, emotional instability, scattered thinking, anger outbursts, and occasional paranoid ideation. The patient had a history of alcohol abuse and bulimia. She was raised in an orphanage and foster homes because her parents were unable to take care of her. She reported that she was sexually abused by her foster father who was an alcoholic. She denied drug abuse. Her biological mother suffered from depression. The patient denied a history of major medical problems.

Axis II Diagnosis: Dependent personality disorder with borderline features

Axis I Diagnosis: Major depression, severe, single episode

Current Treatment:
1. venlafaxine 50 mg BID
2. risperidone 0.5 mg HS
3. Alprazolam 0.25 mg TID
4. psychotherapy (infrequently)

Treatment Course: The patient was hospitalized initially and discharged after stabilizing on nortriptyline 100 mg HS, buspirone 10 mg TID, and lorazepam 1 mg HS. They were eventually discontinued in favor of her current medications, which have been very effective in controlling Axis I and most of the Axis II symptoms. She has been functioning fairly well for approximately the last two years on this combination of medications. She reported that she has felt the most stable emotionally on these medications and would like to stay on them indefinitely.

Comments: Patients who are brought up in an unstable home environment, as was this patient, remain emotionally fragile and vulnerable for most of their lives. While the medications keep them from being acutely symptomatic, the basic vulnerability and dependency symptoms are unlikely to disappear completely. A breakup in a relationship or a major interpersonal conflict will be sufficient for Axis I symptoms to emerge despite the patient being on medication. Patients with Axis II disorders should be maintained on an effective medication long-term for achieving the best outcome.

Case #40

Presenting Symptoms: The patient was a 32-year-old female, with complaints of depressed mood, anxiety, feelings of hopelessness, irritability, frequent crying, excessive emotional sensitivity, insomnia, and hyperphagia. Since early adulthood she had experienced symptoms such as fear of abandonment, excessive reliance on others in making decisions, difficulty asserting herself for fear of disapproval, and poor self-confidence. She relied on her parents or her boyfriend to give direction to her life. The patient's history was obtained from the patient and her parents, who were present during the first office visit. She denied drug and alcohol abuse, smoking, and caffeine intake. She was taking trazodone 150 mg HS (prescribed by her primary care physician), which was not effective. Both parents suffered from depression. Her mother was taking nortriptyline. Medical history is significant for back pain, obesity, and carpal tunnel syndrome. She had been taking an oral contraceptive. Thyroid profile was within normal limits.

Axis II Diagnosis: Dependent personality disorder

Axis I Diagnosis: Major depression, moderate, single episode
Dysthymia

Current Treatment:
1. paroxetine 20 mg AM
2. risperidone 0.5 mg HS
3. temazepam 15 mg HS
4. trazodone 25 mg HS
5. psychotherapy

Treatment Course: The patient was started first on fluoxetine, which had to be discontinued due to excessive restlessness and sweating. She was switched to paroxetine, which did not cause sweating. The patient described a recent episode of extreme fright and helplessness when she could not find her mother for a few minutes in a grocery store. This indicated an almost childlike dependency which is regressive for a 32-year-old woman. Risperidone 0.5 mg was added with marked improvement in her tendency to become overwhelmingly fearful when alone. Trazodone 25 mg and temazepam were prescribed to treat insomnia.

Comments: There was marked improvement in this patient's abandonment fears, anxiety, and overwhelming dependency needs after the addition of a very low dose of risperidone. It is my opinion that extreme fear and dependency respond to low doses of antipsychotics whereas depressive symptoms and milder dependency symptoms respond to antidepressants alone. Dependent personality disorder typically comes to clinical attention due to depression or anxiety precipitated by complications arising from dysfunctional dependency needs and conflicts.

Chapter 11

Obsessive-Compulsive Personality Disorder

The *DSM-IV* criteria for diagnosis of obsessive-compulsive personality disorder are as follows.

DSM-IV *CRITERIA AND SYMPTOM CORRELATES*

A pervasive pattern of preoccupation with orderliness, perfectionism, and mental and interpersonal control, at the expense of flexibility, openness, and efficiency, beginning by early adulthood and present in a variety of contexts, as indicated by four (or more) of the following:

1. *Is preoccupied with details, rules, lists, order, organization, or schedules to the extent that the major point of the activity is lost.*
2. *Shows perfectionism that interferes with task completion (e.g., is unable to complete a project because his or her own overly strict standards are not met).*
3. *Is excessively devoted to work and productivity to the exclusion of leisure activities and friendships (not accounted for by obvious economic necessity).*
4. *Is overconscientious, scrupulous, and inflexible about matters of morality, ethics, or values (not accounted for by cultural or religious identification).*

---

5. *Is unable to discard worn-out or worthless objects even when they have no sentimental value.*
6. *Is reluctant to delegate tasks or to work with others unless they submit to exactly his or her way of doing things.*
7. *Adopts a miserly spending style toward both self and others; money is viewed as something to be hoarded for future catastrophes.*
8. *Shows rigidity and stubbornness.*

The apparent symptom correlates that are possibly responsive to currently available medications are listed in Table 11.1.

From a practical psychopharmacological treatment standpoint, obsessive-compulsive personality symptoms are best considered a mild form of obsessive-compulsive disorder. There appear to be no qualitative differences between obsessive-compulsive personality disorder and obsessive-compulsive disorder, rather only quantitative differences if clinical observation, clinical judgment, and response to medication are to be trusted. It follows that the pharmacological treatment of obsessive-compulsive personality disorder is similar to the treatment of obsessive-compulsive disorder. Though medications such as clomipramine and all of the serotonergic antidepressants, venlafaxine and nefazodone are variably effective for treatment of obsessive-compulsive disorder, in most cases dosages in the upper levels of the dosage range are needed. Some of the more severe forms of obsessive-compulsive disorder are resistant to complete symptom resolution. Such is not the case with obsessive-compulsive personality disorder, which tends to respond at the lower-range or midrange of dose, and is often more successfully treated. The first-line medications for obsessive-compulsive symptoms, whether they are part of obsessive-compulsive personality disorder, generalized anxiety disorder, depression, schizophrenia, or anxiety, are the serotonergic antidepressants, clomipramine or venlafaxine. Although clomipramine is the most effective medication for the treatment of obsessive-compulsive symptoms, its TCA side effects and greater toxicity in overdose make it a second-line medication compared to serotonergic medications. In treatment-resistant cases, a combination of clomipramine with a serotonergic medication may be attempted, as long as the dosage of clomipramine is lowered to assure that seizure risk is not excessive. Because of concerns regarding sei-

TABLE 11.1. Symptom Correlates for Obsessive-Compulsive Personality Disorder

DSM-IV **Criteria**	**Symptom Correlates**
A pervasive pattern of preoccupation with orderliness, perfectionism, and mental and interpersonal control, at the expense of flexibility, openness, and efficiency, beginning by early adulthood and present in a variety of contexts	obsessions and compulsions
1. Is preoccupied with details, rules, lists, order, organization, or schedules to the extent that the major point of the activity is lost	obsessional features
2. Shows perfectionism that interferes with task completion (e.g., is unable to complete a project because his or her own overly strict standards are not met)	compulsive features
3. Is excessively devoted to work and productivity to the exclusions of leisure activities and friendships (not accounted for by obvious economic necessity)	compulsive features
4. Is overconscientious, scrupulous, and inflexible about matters of morality, ethics, or values (not accounted for by cultural or religious identification)	obsessional features
5. Is unable to discard worn-out or worthless objects even when they have no sentimental value	obsessional features
6. Is reluctant to delegate tasks or to work with others unless they submit to exactly his or her way of doing things	compulsive features
7. Adopts a miserly spending style toward both self and others; money is viewed as something to be hoarded for future catastrophies	obsessional features
8. Shows rigidity and stubbornness	obsessional features

zure, the dosage of clomipramine should not exceed the maximum recommended dose of 250 mg per day in divided doses. If, for a particular patient, dosage above 250 mg per day becomes necessary, seizure prophylaxis using an anticonvulsant medication such as valproate or carbamazepine is recommended. Clomipramine should be relatively contraindicated in patients who have a low threshold for seizures such as patients with brain tumors, acute head injuries, or a history of seizures. For those who can tolerate it, clomipramine as a single medication has shown the best results for treatment of obsessive-compulsive symptoms. The criteria for initiating treatment should be: (1) finding even one obsessive-compulsive feature which is causing distress to the patient or others; and (2) the patient is interested in treatment. The physician should initiate appropriate treatment, regardless of whether or not the patient meets the criteria for obsessive-compulsive disorder and/or obsessive-compulsive personality disorder. Remember, treatment is not predicated on diagnosis, but is aimed at resolving a symptom or symptoms, which are a source of distress or cause dysfunction. In nearly all cases, part of the treatment of obsessive-compulsive symptoms requires the use of medications, with cognitive-behavioral therapy providing additional benefits. Psychotherapeutic approaches have a better chance of significantly improving a patient's condition when given to a patient whose acute symptoms are controlled with medication. Observations from treating many mild to severe obsessive-compulsive symptoms suggest that optimal benefits are obtained by the combined use of medication and psychotherapy, rather than either alone, despite the possibility that isolated research studies might demonstrate that one or the other approach is superior. It is an interesting and not surprising observation that, for the most part, research by a biologically oriented researcher tends to show the superiority of medications, and research by a psychologically oriented researcher shows the superiority of psychological interventions, whereas clinical experience shows that both are beneficial in varying degrees in individual patients, and that optimal treatment is a combination of both approaches. Clomipramine, serotonergic antidepressants, venlafaxine, and nefazodone are beneficial in patients with symptoms or behaviors having an obsessional or compulsive nature, even if the behavior in question is not typically associated with obsessive-compulsive disorder or obsessive-compulsive personality disorder symptoms. Examples include erotomania, body dysmorphic disorder, fixed delusions (as in paranoid disorder), pedophilia, and addictions to substances or to various behaviors, regardless of the diagnosis. These are sometimes referred to as obsessive-compulsive spectrum disorders. For treatment of atypical obsessive-compulsive behavior, the author has found clomipramine to be very effective in the low to medium dosage range (e.g., 50 mg to 150 mg per day in divided doses). The problem behavior might not completely subside, but the intensity of the urge and the frequency tend to decrease, offering better control to the individual patient and some relief to others.

Other combinations of medications that have been found to be effective are serotonergic antidepressants and high potency benzodiazepines such as clonazepam, alprazolam, and lorazepam. Combination treatment is usually attempted only after various single medications are tried individually at the maximum tolerated dose, within the approved dosage range, and are found to be either partially effective or ineffective. Adjunctive medications include lithium, carbamazepine, valproate, trazodone, clonidine, guanfacine, low-dose antipsychotics, buspirone (Buspar), and high-potency benzodiazepines. Low-dose antipsychotics are advisable only in cases where obsessive-compulsive symptoms are so severe that they reach psychotic or regressive proportions; hence, they would not ordinarily be a consideration when dealing with obsessive-compulsive personality disorder where–by definition–the clinician is dealing with relatively milder symptoms that patients have managed to live with for a long time despite being fairly dysfunctional. It is important that patients are told that control of symptoms will enable them to utilize their full intellectual, creative, and occupational potentials, which are suppressed by the various obsessions and compulsions. Such hopeful and encouraging reassurance has the potential to motivate even some of the more ambivalent patients.

The dosages of some of the adjunctive medications are given below:

1. lithium (Eskalith CR 450 mg or Lithobid 300 mg)–600 mg to 900 mg per day in divided doses to obtain a serum level of 0.4 mEq/L to 0.8 mEq/L (For adjunctive uses, there is no need for a higher serum level.)

2. carbamazepine (Tegretol)–300 mg to 600 mg per day in divided doses, to get a serum level between 4.0 mcg/DL and 8.0 mcg/DL
3. valproate–750 mg to 1250 mg per day in divided doses, to achieve a blood level of 40 mcg/L to 80 mcg/L
4. clonazepam–0.5 mg BID, alprazolam–0.5 mg TID, and lorazepam–0.5 mg TID
5. trazodone–50 mg TID
6. clonidine–0.1 mg BID-TID
7. buspirone (Buspar)–20 to 40 mg per day in divided doses
8. antipsychotics should be used as an adjunctive medication at very low doses only if other medications fail and if there is significant improvement, making the risk-benefit ratio favorable. The usual dosage range when used adjunctively is haloperidol 0.5 mg to 2 mg per day as a divided or bedtime dose, or equivalent dosage of another antipsychotic. Among all of the antipsychotics, the author's choice as first-line medications currently are risperidone at 0.5 to 1.5 mg per day in divided or once-a-day dose, olanzapine 2.5 to 5 mg HS, or sertindole 4 to 8 mg HS.

If all of the above medications fail, a trial of an MAOI may be initiated. Coadministration of an MAOI with other antidepressants and buspirone is generally contraindicated.

CLINICAL CASES 41 to 48

Case #41

Presenting Symptoms: The patient was a 57-year-old female, with symptoms consisting of perfectionistic tendencies, obsessive rumination, compulsive arranging and organizing, anxiety, anorexia, and insomnia. The obsessive-compulsive characteristics have been present for as long as she can remember. She also reported episodes of somnambulism. She admitted to a habit of drinking four glasses of wine, smoking two packs of cigarettes, and drinking three cups of coffee daily. She denied any acute precipitants. The patient's medical history was unremarkable.

Axis II Diagnosis: Obsessive-compulsive personality disorder

Axis I Diagnosis: Sleep-walking disorder
Alcohol dependence, mild

Current Treatment: 1. clomipramine 50 mg HS
2. psychotherapy

Treatment Course: Outpatient detoxification using tapering doses of chlordiazepoxide enabled her to safely stop alcohol consumption. Clomipramine was started at 25 mg HS, and increased to 50 mg, which resulted in remarkable improvement in her obsessive-compulsive symptoms in addition to eliminating the sleep-walking.

Comments: Although clomipramine is the best antiobsessional medication currently available, it has the disadvantage of possessing TCA side effects. Hence SSRIs, which have a favorable side effect profile, are generally preferred as first-line medications for treatment of obsessive-compulsive symptoms. A low dose of clomipramine (25 to 100 mg per day) may be safely tried in patients with obsessive-compulsive symptoms, anxiety symptoms, insomnia, and anorexia. Clomipramine was chosen for a first trial in this patient for the following reasons:

- The patient had obsessive-compulsive personality disorder symptoms.
- Somnambulism typically occurs in slow-wave sleep stages three and four (TCAs decrease the intensity of slow-wave sleep).
- The patient complained of symptoms such as anxiety, insomnia, and anorexia.

Fortunately, the patient tolerated the medication well and had excellent results.

Generally, fairly low doses of antiobsessional medication are sufficient for treatment of obsessive-compulsive personality disorder, as compared to obsessive-compulsive disorder. For practical treatment purposes, obsessive-compulsive personality disorder may be considered a very mild form of obsessive-compulsive disorder. It is a common clinical observation that mild symptoms respond to doses lower than that typically used for treating severe symptoms.

Medication response is not an all-or-nothing phenomenon, but occurs in a gradient. The general dosage ranges for obsessive-compulsive personality disorder and obsessive-compulsive disorder are listed in Table 11.2.

Since alcohol has sedative properties, it is commonly abused as a form of "self-medication," particularly by patients with anxiety disorders including obsessive-compulsive disorder, as was observed in this case. It is possible that this patient's sleepwalking resolved due to abstention from alcohol.

TABLE 11.2. Dosage Ranges of Medication to Treat Obsessive-Compulsive and Obsessive-Compulsive Personality Disorders

Obsessive-Compulsive Personality Disorder		**Obsessive-Compulsive Disorder**	
clomipramine	25 - 100 mg/day	clomipramine	50 - 250 mg/day
fluoxetine	25 - 40 mg/day	fluoxetine	40 - 100 mg/day*
fluvoxamine	50 - 100 mg/day	fluvoxamine	100 - 300 mg/day
sertraline	50 - 100 mg/day	sertraline	100 - 300 mg/day*
paroxetine	20 - 40 mg/day	paroxetine	30 - 90 mg/day*
venlafaxine	25 - 50 mg TID	venlafaxine	50 - 125 mg TID

*Maximum manufacturer's recommended dose for fluoxetine is 80 mg, sertraline 200 mg, and paroxetine 60 mg per day.

Case #42

Presenting Symptoms: The patient was a 49-year-old female, with complaints of obsessive fear of losing close friends or relatives, perfectionistic tendencies, excessive orderliness, anxiety, somatic preoccupation, vague fears, excessive worrying, depressed mood, anhedonia, and restless sleep. These symptoms had been present since early adulthood, but had worsened during the last two to three years without any identifiable precipitants. She denied drug and alcohol abuse, smoking, and caffeine intake. The patient had been taking alprazolam 0.5 mg BID, prescribed by her primary care physician. She had taken chlordiazepoxide many years ago. The patient's mother suffered from depression. The patient is on atenolol 50 mg daily for mitral valve prolapse, and on ranitidine 150 mg BID for peptic ulcer.

Axis II Diagnosis: Obsessive-compulsive personality disorder

Current Treatment: 1. paroxetine 20 mg HS
2. alprazolam 0.25 mg PRN for anxiety

Treatment Course: The patient was given paroxetine 20 mg AM, which improved all of the presenting symptoms. Alprazolam was decreased to 0.25 mg BID for several weeks, and then changed to PRN use. Since paroxetine caused mild sedation during day time, the schedule was switched to bedtime, with further improvement in sleep and in daytime alertness. The patient has been on paroxetine now for two years and wants to continue the medication indefinitely.

Comments: Whether this is a case of mild obsessive-compulsive disorder or obsessive-compulsive personality disorder, the treatment is the same. It is often difficult to distinguish between obsessive-compulsive personality disorder and mild cases of obsessive-compulsive disorder; therefore, reliance on symptoms is the primary determinant in terms of selecting medication. Antiobsessional medications are generally more effective for symptoms of obsessive-compulsive personality disorder than for severe cases of obsessive-compulsive disorder. Strictly from a psychopharmacological standpoint, obsessive-compulsive personality disorders are conceptualized as a mild form of chronic obsessive-compulsive disorder and are eminently treatable using clomipramine or SSRIs.

Obsessive-compulsive symptoms nearly always coexist with depressive and anxiety symptoms. Fortunately, antiobsessional medications nicely control depression and anxiety, making separate treatment usually unnecessary.

Since personality symptoms are chronic in nature in the sense that the symptoms have been present for many years, it may be necessary to continue maintenance medication treatment for several years prior to discontinuation. Many patients realize such relief from their symptoms that they request continuation on the medication indefinitely.

Case #43

Presenting Symptoms: The patient was a 35-year-old male, with symptoms consisting of depressed mood, insomnia, loss of appetite, loss of weight, crying episodes, feelings of hopelessness, anergia, irritability, and anhedonia, precipitated by separation from his lover. The patient described a personality pattern characterized by symptoms such as perfectionistic tendencies, compulsive organizing and arranging, excessive worrying, and stubborn attitudes. He denied drug and alcohol abuse, smoking, and caffeine intake. His mother suffered from depression.

Axis II Diagnosis: Obsessive-compulsive personality disorder

Axis I Diagnosis: Major depression, moderate, single episode

Current Treatment:
1. paroxetine 20 mg AM
2. doxepin 10 mg HS
3. temazepam 7.5 mg HS
4. psychotherapy

Treatment Course: Significant improvement in both Axis I and Axis II symptoms were reported by the patient two weeks after starting medications as listed above; hence, medication dosage adjustments were not necessary. The patient is currently maintained on these medications with a nearly complete resolution of the symptoms.

Comments: Treatment that takes into consideration both Axis I and Axis II symptoms strives to resolve all of the presenting and underlying symptoms; thus, the choice of medication should not only be based on the presenting symptoms (usually, but not necessarily, Axis I symptoms), but also on underlying personality characteristics. A comprehensive treatment should address all of the symptoms.

This patient's symptoms and medications may be grouped as follows:

Symptom Group	Medication Class	Specific Medication
Depressive symptoms	antidepressant	paroxetine 20 mg AM
Obsessive-compulsive personality symptoms	antiobsessional	paroxetine 20 mg AM
Marked anorexia	TCA	doxepin 10 mg HS
Insomnia	sedative-hypnotic	temazepam 7.5 mg HS doxepin 10 mg HS

Since paroxetine has both antidepressant and antiobsessional effects, it efficiently treats two major symptom groups. Doxepin has overlapping effects on stimulating appetite and on enhancing sleep. The use of doxepin made it possible to keep the dose of temazepam extremely low at 7.5 mg. Without doxepin, the temazepam dose most likely would have been higher. Given the tolerance, habituation, and dependence risks associated with sedative-hypnotics, it is important to keep dosages low. This can be accomplished by using adjunctive sleep aids such as TCAs with sedating effects.

Case #44

Presenting Symptoms: The patient was a 49-year-old male, with symptoms consisting of anhedonia, anxiety, depressed mood, perfectionistic tendencies, excessive preoccupation with work, stubbornness, and preoccupation with orderliness. The patient reported that most of the above characteristics had been present since his late twenties. He denied drug and alcohol abuse. He reported smoking two packs of cigarettes per day and drinking ten cups of coffee daily. His depression and anxiety recently emerged due to marital conflicts. The patient had had psychotherapy intermittently in the past. He denied a family history of psychiatric disorders. His medical history was significant for benign prostatic hypertrophy for which he was taking terazosin (Hytrin).

Axis II Diagnosis: Obsessive-compulsive personality disorder

Axis I Diagnosis: Caffeine-induced anxiety disorder

Current Treatment:
1. fluoxetine 20 mg AM
2. decrease coffee intake to two cups of coffee daily

Treatment Course: Fluoxetine 20 mg AM was started at the first visit. Depressive and anxiety symptoms, and chronic obsessive-compulsive personality symptoms showed satisfactory improvement.

Comments: This is another case example of the effectiveness of SSRIs in the treatment of Axis II obsessive-compulsive personality disorder symptoms.

Case #45

Presenting Symptoms: The patient was a 27-year-old male, whose symptoms consisted of counting rituals, compulsive cleaning, perfectionistic tendencies, depressed mood, feelings of hopelessness, rigid attitudes, anergia, severe insomnia, anxiety, and excessive devotion to work. Most of the above symptoms had been present since his early twenties. Depressive symptoms worsened recently due to marital conflicts. He denied drug and alcohol abuse, smoking, and caffeine intake. The patient's older sister had a diagnosis of depression. He denied major medical problems.

Axis II Diagnosis: Obsessive-compulsive personality disorder

Axis I Diagnosis: Adjustment disorder with depressed mood
Consider obsessive-compulsive disorder, mild

Current Treatment:
1. fluoxetine 60 mg AM
2. trazodone 100 mg AM
3. temazepam 7.5 mg HS PRN insomnia
4. continue psychotherapy

Treatment Course: The patient was started on fluoxetine 20 mg AM, trazodone 50 mg HS, and temazepam 7.5 mg HS. Some improvement was reported when seen two weeks later. The dose of fluoxetine was gradually increased to his current dose of 60 mg AM over a period of ten weeks. Since trazodone 50 mg HS did not fully treat insomnia, the dose was increased to 100 mg HS with excellent results. The patient reported marked improvement not only in his depression but also in his obsessive-compulsive tendencies.

Comments: This is another simple case that illustrates the common observation that Axis I symptoms such as depressed mood, anxiety, and insomnia are the presenting symptoms and that it is rare that a patient will seek psychiatric help simply to manage a personality disorder. However, as illustrated in this case, it is important to diagnose the personality disorder, if present, so that the most effective treatment can be recommended. For instance, if the diagnostic evaluation focused only on Axis I symptoms, the choice of an antidepressant might be any of the antidepressants, including TCAs, MAOIs, or bupropion. It is possible for a TCA or MAOI to treat the depressive and anxiety symptoms as effectively as the SSRIs. However, a TCA or MAOI is not the drug of choice for treating obsessive-compulsive symptoms (except for clomipramine). SSRIs and clomipramine are the drugs of choice for treating obsessive-compulsive symptoms with or without accompanying depression and anxiety. It is clear that the identification of a personality disorder has practical treatment implications in modern psychiatric practice, whereas prior to 1990, the diagnosis of a personality disorder did not have much practical significance as it related to pharmacological intervention.

It is an increasingly common clinical observation that most Axis II symptoms are as amenable to treatment as Axis I symptoms if aggressively treated. This gives us hope that one day there will be medications to treat the superego defects seen among antisocial personality disorders, which currently manifest some of the most treatment-resistant symptoms in psychopharmacological practice.

Case #46

Presenting Symptoms: The patient was a 58-year-old male, with complaints of anxiety, vague fears, insomnia, anxiety attacks, excessive meticulousness and punctuality, perfectionistic tendencies, excessive worrying, obsessive preoccupation with a fear of dying, depressed mood, and compulsive arranging. He reported that the obsessive-compulsive tendencies had been present for more than 30 years. He had previously been tried on doxepin, clomipramine, and alprazolam, which were not quite effective. He denied drug and alcohol abuse and smoking. He drank one cup of coffee daily. The patient denied a family history of psychiatric disorders. He also denied any major medical problems.

Axis II Diagnosis:	Obsessive-compulsive personality disorder
Axis I Diagnosis:	Generalized anxiety disorder Consider panic disorder
Current Treatment:	1. paroxetine 45 mg AM 2. clonazepam 0.25 mg BID 3. Triavil 2/10 HS 4. referral for psychotherapy

Treatment Course: Other medications tried at various times as an outpatient were buspirone, fluoxetine, diazepam, risperidone, venlafaxine, amitriptyline, and fluvoxamine. None of these were fully effective. Eventually, the patient responded well to the present combination of medications which he has been taking for the last year.

The patient experienced remarkable improvement of anxiety symptoms and of obsessive-compulsive symptoms.

Comments: The doses of clonazepam and Triavil are extremely low; yet, the addition of these medications to the primary medication (paroxetine) had a noticeably beneficial effect and resulted in overall improvement. Antipsychotics are generally not indicated for anxiety disorders or for nonpsychotic symptoms. However, there are some patients whose anxiety symptoms respond nicely to low doses of antipsychotics, but not to benzodiazepines, for unknown reasons. A possibility exists that these patients could have a mild alteration in the balance of the dopamine neurotransmitter system that manifests clinically as anxiety rather than psychosis. Generally, very low doses of antipsychotics may be tried in these patients as a last resort, after trying various antidepressants, antianxiety medications, and buspirone. If, however, a patient is to be maintained on the antipsychotic for more than three to four months, it is important to inform the patient of the risk of tardive dyskinesia (in the case of elderly patients, tardive dyskinesia can be a risk after one to two months if the doses of antipsychotics are fairly high). Risperidonem, olanzapine, and sertindole probably have a decreased risk of inducing tardive dyskinesia compared to traditional antipsychotics. Clozapine is not known to cause tardive dyskinesia.

Case #47

Presenting Symptoms: The patient was a 25-year-old male, whose symptoms consisted of perfectionistic tendencies, rigid and concrete thinking, excessive preoccupation with details, obsessive rumination, anxiety, irritability, and insomnia. The obsessional features had been present since his late teens. He had been taking fluoxetine 20 mg AM for one year when first seen at the office. He denied drug and alcohol abuse, smoking, and caffeine intake. His uncle had had a "nervous breakdown." His medical history was significant for cerebral palsy and mild scoliosis.

Axis II Diagnosis: Obsessive-compulsive personality disorder

Current Treatment: fluoxetine 40 mg AM

Treatment Course: The dose of fluoxetine was increased to 40 mg AM at the first office visit. The patient reported further improvement in obsessional symptoms when seen two weeks later. He has continued to function well for the last six months.

Comments: SSRIs and clomipramine are effective for the treatment of symptoms of obsessive-compulsive personality disorders, and hence should be considered for the treatment of all patients with distressing obsessive-compulsive personality symptoms even if the symptoms do not meet the full *DSM-IV* criteria.

Case #48

Presenting Symptoms: The patient was a 27-year-old male, with complaints of frequent panic attacks, depressive episodes, feelings of hopelessness, insomnia, obsessive rumination, perfectionistic tendencies, excessive preoccupation with work, anxiety, mild compulsive cleaning, and mood swings. He denied drug and alcohol abuse, smoking, and caffeine intake. He had been placed on imipramine, clonazepam, and sertraline in the past, with no significant effect. The patient's father had a diagnosis of depression. The patient was taking atenolol 50 mg for hypertension.

Axis II Diagnosis: Obsessive-compulsive personality disorder

Axis I Diagnosis: Panic disorder
Dysthymia

Current Treatment:
1. fluvoxamine 100 mg AM and 200 mg HS
2. alprazolam 0.25 mg QID
3. referred for counseling

Treatment Course: Various medications including fluoxetine and paroxetine were not effective. Marked improvement was seen with fluvoxamine, which was started at 100 mg HS, and gradually increased to the current dose. He is seen once every three months for medication management.

Comments: In most cases, an effective medication or combination of medications can be found if the physician is determined and if the patient is cooperative. Because of the favorable side effect profile of SSRIs, my approach is to place the patient on a trial of SSRIs until most choices are exhausted. With the numerous choices of SSRIS, one of them is likely to be effective. Although fluvoxamine is only approved for the treatment of obsessive compulsive disorder, its actions are like other SSRIs and it is effective for the SSRI indications such as depression and anxiety. The combination of fluvoxamine and alprazolam resolved this patient's Axis I and Axis II symptoms. Perfectionistic tendencies, compulsive tendencies, and excessive preoccupation with work improved satisfactorily.

Chapter 12

Personality Disorder, Not Otherwise Specified (NOS)

Personality Disorder, NOS is the diagnosis used when the patient presents with features of more than one specific personality disorder that do not meet the full criteria for any one of the personality disorders but cause clinically significant distress or impairment in functioning. It is also known as "Mixed Personality Disorder" or "Personality Disorder with Mixed Features." Examples include features of passive-aggressive, depressive, hypomanic, anxious, and self-defeating personality disorders, which are not currently recognized *DSM-IV* diagnoses.

Most personality disorders have features that are characteristics of more than one personality disorder. It is not common to see patients in clinical practice who precisely fit the *DSM-IV* criteria set for a specific personality disorder. In the majority of cases, different personality disorder features at varying levels coexist along with Axis I symptoms. The concept of symptom-focused treatment is particularly relevant in the treatment of personality disorder, NOS because of the lack of diagnostic focus by definition.

CLINICAL CASE 49

Case #49

Presenting Symptoms: The patient was a 49-year-old female, whose symptoms consisted of depressed mood, frequent crying, feelings of hopelessness, inability to function at work, disorganized thinking, severe anxiety, mood instability, grandiosity, hypomanic episodes, initial insomnia, episodes of intense anger, paranoid fears, labile affect, perfectionistic tendencies, and social anxiety. Most of the symptoms at less severity had been present for the last 20 to 25 years, as reported by the patient. She had a history of alcohol and drug abuse, but had abstained for the past five years. The symptoms were recently exacerbated due to conflicts with her boss. She had intermittently received psychotherapy in the past. She was taking estrogen supplements.

Axis II Diagnosis: Personality disorder, NOS

Axis I Diagnosis: Major depression, moderate, recurrent
Consider bipolar II

Current Treatment:
1. fluoxetine 20 mg AM
2. risperidone 0.5 mg HS
3. zolpidem 5 mg HS PRN insomnia
4. psychotherapy

Treatment Course: Venlafaxine, bupropion, valproate, carbamazepine, and paroxetine were tried but were discontinued either due to side effects or lack of effect. The current combination of fluoxetine and risperidone has significantly improved the depressive symptoms as well as most of the personality disorder symptoms.

Comments: In actual practice, a diagnosis of "Personality Disorder, NOS" is not uncommon because many patients present with symptoms of more than one personality disorder but do not meet the full criteria for any one personality disorder. In these instances, as is true of all diagnoses, the presence of specific symptoms determine the choice of medications. Although this patient had a variety of symptoms, fluoxetine and a very low dose of risperidone effectively controlled most of the symptoms. If there is no emergency, medications are best added sequentially so that the need for adding various medications can be assessed during the course of several months, when there is the opportunity to evaluate the effects of the existing medication. However, in a psychiatric emergency as in the treatment of a manic or highly agitated patient, several medications are given concurrently to achieve rapid control of symptoms.

Chapter 13

Personality Change Due to a General Medical Condition (AXIS I)

Personality change due to a general medical condition is commonly known as organic personality disorder or organic personality syndrome, and is coded on Axis I, *not* on Axis II. This condition represents a personality change that is precipitated by the direct physiological effects of a medical condition.

The general mechanism by which these general medical conditions precipitate a personality change is by affecting the functions of the brain, directly or indirectly, in nearly all cases. The common general medical conditions that can lead to a personality change are listed below.

COMMON GENERAL MEDICAL CONDITIONS THAT CAN LEAD TO PERSONALITY CHANGE

concussion
epilepsy
Parkinson's disease
stroke
head trauma
endocrine abnormalities
neurosyphilis (not common in the United States currently)
encephalitis (including HIV-related)
Huntington's disease
multiple sclerosis
brain tumor

brain injury
systemic lupus erythematosis
cerebrovascular disease
CNS infections

Patient history, physical examination, or laboratory findings are relied upon to determine whether or not the general medical condition is etiologically related to the personality change. A temporal association between the onset of the general medical condition and the personality change is usually sufficient to suggest the etiology. The onset of the personality change may be immediate or gradual. In cases where objective anatomical or biochemical lesions are not evident, as in the case of a closed head injury (e.g., concussion, contusion, etc.), the patient's history is of singular importance. Occasionally, neuropsychological and psychological tests offer standardized information. However, absence of test findings indicative of personality change or of abnormalities does not rule out the possibility that the personality change was due to the general medical condition. The finding of a personality change remains a clinical finding and should be made by a qualified clinician after taking into consideration all available data. The fact that personality change can occur due to medical conditions offers further support to the author's opinion that Axis II personality disorders may in fact also have varying degrees of biological bases.

In most cases, the personality change (due to a general medical condition) consists of a clinically significant exacerbation of previous personality tendencies rather than emergence of completely new personality characteristics. For example, an individual who had obsessional or paranoid tendencies could become markedly more symptomatic due to a concussion, encephalitis, epilepsy, stroke, brain tumor, or one of the other general medical conditions, as illustrated by Case #50. The primary diagnostic criteria for personality change due to a general medical condition based on *DSM-IV* are as follows:

1. A persistent personality disturbance that is a change from the premorbid personality pattern.
2. The personality change is etiologically related to the direct physiological consequence of a general medical condition as

evidenced by data from the history, physical examination, or laboratory findings.

3. The personality change leads to clinically significant distress or impairment in social, occupational, or other important areas of functioning.

The acute effects of general medical conditions or common clinical characteristics of degenerative diseases are excluded from the diagnostic criteria. For example, the acute behavioral manifestations of delirium or the emergence of paranoia associated with dementia are not included in the criteria for personality change due to a general medical condition. Various symptom characteristics that represent the personality change can predominate in the clinical presentation. The following are the main subtypes listed in *DSM-IV*:

Subtype	Predominant Features
Labile Type	affective lability
Disinhibited Type	poor impulse control
Aggressive Type	aggressive behavior
Apathetic Type	apathy and indifference
Paranoid Type	paranoia or suspiciousness
Combined Type	combination of various characteristics
Unspecified Type	other features

Psychiatric treatment (assuming the general medical conditions have been optimally addressed medically) consists as always of identification of specific symptoms and initiation of treatment to alleviate the severity of symptoms. Possible medication options for each of the subtypes are listed below. Combinations of medications may be necessary for optimal control of symptoms if a single medication is not effective.

Subtype	Preferred Medication Options
Labile Type	antidepressants mood stabilizers

Disinhibited Type	antidepressants (low dose, sedating) antipsychotics, clonidine, guanfacine, beta-blockers, stimulants
Aggressive Type	beta-blockers, clonidine, guanfacine, antidepressants (SSRIs preferred), buspirone, antipsychotics
Apathetic Type	stimulating antidepressants stimulants
Paranoid Type	antipsychotics
Combined Type	combinations

Frequently, a sequential trial of various medications from different classes is necessary to arrive at a medication or a combination of medications to control symptoms. If the general medical condition improves, a concomitant improvement in the personality disturbance is expected, resulting in the need for a decrease in the dose of medications or the elimination of medications. Generally, psychotropic medications are employed in relatively low doses in patients who have a general medical condition because these patients tend to be more sensitive to psychotropic medications than patients without a general medical condition.

CLINICAL CASE 50

Case #50

Presenting Symptoms: The patient was a 60-year-old male. He was involuntarily brought by police and admitted to the inpatient psychiatric unit after he became assaultive toward his wife, destructive to property, hostile, and agitated. Several months prior to his psychiatric hospitalization, he had suffered a cerebrovascular accident (CVA), which damaged the speech center causing expressive aphasia. Since the stroke, he had been exhibiting violent rages, paranoid ideation, crying episodes, and extreme mood swings. He also suffered from anorexia and insomnia. His wife reported that he had had an irritable and angry temperament all of his adult years and that the stroke made his anger and moodiness even worse. However, rage attacks, assaultive behavior, and paranoia were not present prior to his stroke. He had been in the habit of drinking two to three beers daily. Alcohol worsened the mood lability. He denied drug abuse. He smoked one pack of cigarettes daily, and drank one to two cups of regular coffee daily. The patient's medical history was unremarkable, except as described above. He denied previous psychiatric treatment and denied a family history of psychiatric disorders, except that the patient's father was described as "hot-tempered."

Current Diagnosis: Personality change due to CVA, combined type (Axis I)

Other possible diagnoses:

Alcohol abuse
Dysthymia
Bipolar disorder, NOS

Current Treatment:

1. fluoxetine 60 mg AM
2. carbamazepine 200 mg TID
3. Triavil 4/10 HS (brand name for a fixed ratio tablet containing perphenazine and amitriptyline)

Treatment Course: The patient's agitation was controlled using haloperidol 5 mg IM and lorazepam 1 mg IM in the hospital. After the first dose of IM medication, he became cooperative and was started on fluoxetine 20 mg AM, carbamazepine 200 mg BID, lorazepam 0.5 mg TID, and Triavil 2/10 HS. The dose of fluoxetine was increased to 40 mg AM after seven days. The dose of carbamazepine was increased to 200 mg TID to achieve a therapeutic serum level. Lorazepam was tapered off prior to discharge. The patient was discharged after nine days and before optimal results were achieved because he refused to stay longer. It was only with considerable persuasion and threats of separation by his wife that he had stayed for the nine days. When seen in the office after three weeks, his wife reported continuing mood disturbance, although not as severe as prior to his hospitalization. The fluoxetine dose was increased to 60 mg in the morning. At the next follow-up appointment, his wife reported improvement in the patient's irritability and anger outbursts, but complained of suspiciousness. The dose of Triavil was increased to 4/10 at bedtime. A month later, the patient's symptoms had improved to the point that family members were able to tolerate him. He is now seen in the office every six months. According to his wife, he still drinks one to two beers a day, despite the recommendation to abstain. Psychiatric treatment has also made it possible for him to cooperate with his speech therapist without becoming frustrated and hostile.

Comments: Prior to his stroke, this patient may have had dysthymia, cyclothymia, or a personality disorder and probably mild alcohol abuse. His temperament placed a great deal of stress on his family. The CVA significantly worsened the existing symptoms to the point that he was out of control. The mechanism of exacerbation may be related to the disinhibitory effects of the stroke or the extreme helplessness and frustration related to the motor sequelae of the stroke, or both. Regardless of the etiology, symptom control was necessary. From his wife's description of his premorbid personality, it is likely that he would have benefitted from an antidepressant even before the stroke, particularly one of the selective serotonin reuptake inhibitors (SSRIs). Paranoia was a feature that appeared to have emerged after the stroke. Assaultiveness and rage attacks may be considered a quantitatively more severe form of hostility, anger outbursts, and irritability, which were preexisting features. The patient's wife had considered divorce many years earlier because of difficulty coping with his temper but continued in the marriage for the sake of their children. There were four overlapping symptoms that were thought to respond optimally to four separate medications in this patient.

Main Target Symptoms	Medication
mood—anger, irritability, crying	fluoxetine
extreme mood swings	carbamazepine
paranoia, assaultiveness	perphenazine
anorexia, insomnia	amitriptyline

Some of the medications have overlapping effects on symptoms. It would have been ideal to have been able to place this patient on systematic and sequential medication trials in the safe setting of a hospital. Given the increasingly constraining limitations on hospitalization and length of treatment, such an approach is no longer realistic. Third-party payers do not approve lengthy hospital stays; patients may not be able to afford long hospitalizations; the longer the hospitalization, the more the patients' lives are disrupted. It is common knowledge that antidepressants take from 10 to 30 days for optimal effect. In most cases, the number of days in the hospital is not sufficient for making a definitive determination as to whether or not the antidepressant is truly effective at the starting dose. Out of practical necessity, the clinician has to make a judgment and provide a treatment that will control symptoms rapidly. Although all physicians make judgments, the task is more subjective in the specialty of psychiatry and hence more dependent on the particular psychiatric clinician's understanding of the patient's problems. This is in significant contrast to most other medical specialties, where radiographs, and laboratory tests such as blood chemistry and microbiological tests provide more objective and definitive information, enabling the physician to institute specific treatment with a very high degree of confidence and prognostic certainty. The use of combinations of medications is therefore necessary for rapid symptom control. It is my view that the judicious use of medication combinations, based on an understanding of which medications treat which target symptoms, improves treatment outcome and maximizes the patient's overall functioning, without causing overmedication. It is possible, but unlikely, that this patient could have done as well on a single medication. When I recently suggested to the family that we taper off one or more medications sequentially to see if fewer medications would sustain the improvement, the family ardently requested that we not change what was "working." Amitriptyline is probably not necessary at this point. Perphenazine could also be discontinued or the dose decreased without adverse consequences. Fluoxetine is the primary medication required in this patient at this time, with carbamazepine helping adjunctively. If an antipsychotic is needed, risperidone, which was not available at the time the patient was hospitalized, would have been the first-line antipsychotic. Olanzapine, a recently introduced atypical antipsychotic, would also be an excellent choice. Any of the SSRIs would have done an equally good job; I happened to choose fluoxetine. Paroxetine, nefazodone, mirtazapine, venlafaxine, and fluvoxamine were not available at the time. Similarly, valproic acid would have been a reasonable choice. The important concept is that different medications were chosen to address different target symptoms. The specific medication under each class of medications is not as important as the choice of medication class. The dosages should also reflect the purpose. For example, amitriptyline at low doses can provide appetite stimulation, improved sleep, and anticholinergic effects (which are beneficial to patients on high-potency antipsychotics) but is without antidepressant effects. At high doses, amitriptyline acts as an antidepressant with perhaps excessive side effects. Both the choice of medication and the dosage are important for achieving the right "balance," whereby all the symptoms are under satisfactory control without side effects.

PART II:
CLINICAL PROFILES OF SELECTED PSYCHIATRIC DRUGS

Chapter 14

Clinical Profiles of Selected New Generation Antidepressants

BUPROPION (WELLBUTRIN) AND BUPROPION SR (WELLBUTRIN SR)

Bupropion is a norepinephrinergic antidepressant with mild dopaminergic properties and a half-life of approximately ten hours. It is metabolized by the liver and primarily excreted by the kidneys. The dosage range is between 100 mg and 450 mg. The maximum single dose is 150 mg and the maximum total daily dose is 450 mg. It is available in 75 mg and 100 mg tablets. Though it is not scored, it can be easily cut using a pill splitter to obtain lower doses. Several elderly patients have shown adequate response at a dose as low as 50 mg daily.

Bupropion is particularly effective for patients presenting with symptoms such as anergia or decreased energy, apathy, psychomotor retardation, poor concentration, anhedonia, loss of interest in activities that were once enjoyable, and depressed mood. It is also a good choice for patients who have depression associated with bipolar disorder, hypomania, and cyclothymia, since it may not increase "cycling" as frequently as other antidepressants, as well as for depressed patients with attention deficit symptoms.

If the highest single dose of 150 mg is used, a dosing interval of six hours is recommended to decrease the risk of seizure due to peak drug levels that can lower the seizure threshold. Since bupropion decreases the seizure threshold at twice the rate of other antidepressants, the single maximum dose limit of 150 mg and daily total maximum limit of 450 mg should be strictly followed. The estimate of seizures reported in the PDR is 4 per 1,000 for bupropion and approximately 2 per 1000 for other antidepressants. Bupropion is started in outpatients at 75 to 100 mg po AM and at noon for one week, and if there is no adequate response, increased to 100 mg po AM, at noon, and at 5 p.m. for one week. If side effects such as anxiety, headache, or insomnia develop, symptomatic treatment is appropriate. For example, for anxiety, lorazepam 0.5 mg po up to TID, or alprazolam 0.25 mg to 0.5 mg po up to TID may be used. For insomnia, lorazepam 0.5 mg po hs, zolpidem 5 mg to 10 mg po hs, or temazepam 15 mg to 30 mg po hs may be tried.

If, after one week, there is no adequate response to bupropion 100 mg po TID, and if side effects are not significant, the dosage may be increased to 150 mg po TID with specific advice to take the doses with a minimum six-hour interval between doses. The last dose should be taken before 6 or 7 p.m. to decrease the chance that bupropion will interfere with sleep. When side effects become intolerable and cannot be managed, further dosage increase should not be attempted and consideration should be given to discontinuing the medication.

Since bupropion is not available in generic form at the time of this writing, a patient who takes 150 mg po TID will need to take two 75 mg tablets to get a 150 mg dose, needing a total of six tablets a day. At 60 cents a pill, the total daily cost will be approximately $3.60, and the monthly cost at approximately $108.

A history of seizures and bulimia/anorexia are contraindications to prescribing bupropion. Patients taking bupropion should be made aware of seizure precautions, dosage limits, and the necessity of avoiding alcohol. They should also be instructed to avoid activities that could decrease seizure threshold, such as sleep deprivation. The fact that the patient was instructed on the above precautions should be noted on the chart. Though seizure by itself is not a serious incident–it may even improve depression–it can be dangerous and fatal, depending on the context in which it occurs; hence, seizure risk should be taken seriously. If the patient is not warned of the dosage limits and of the relatively higher risk of seizure while taking bupropion, the physician may be held liable should injury occur due to seizure. Many patients, if they forget a dose, will double the next dose to catch up. A patient taking bupropion 100 mg po BID, TID, or QID should be *specifically* advised *not* to take two tablets together to "catch up," since 200 mg dose exceeds the single dose maximum of 150 mg.

Bupropion has been successfully used for treatment of attention deficit hyperactivity disorder (ADHD) at generally lower doses compared to the dosage for treatment of depression. Its energizing and antidepressant properties might possibly be exploited to assist patients coping with nicotine withdrawal in the context of participation in a multidisciplinary smoking cessation program. The sustained-release formulation of bupropion is probably a safer option for this purpose, compared to the regular (immediate-release) formulation.

Bupropion is remarkably devoid of any deleterious effects on libido or sexual performance. Given the high prevalence of sexual side effects associated with serotonergic antidepressants and MAOIs, and the moderate prevalence with TCAs, bupropion has a distinct advantage in this respect. I have found occasional success in partially restoring sexual function and libido in patients by adding a low dose of bupropion (at doses of 75 mg to 100 mg po BID) to a serotonergic antidepressant. However, the success rate of this intervention is not high. Bupropion can also be adjunctively added at low doses if the primary antidepressant fails to improve anergia. It should be remembered that the addition of bupropion has the potential to decrease seizure threshold, especially if the patient is on a TCA, which can independently decrease seizure threshold relatively more than serotonergic medications. Hence, the dose of bupropion should not exceed 200 mg per day in divided doses, and the dose of the primary antidepressant should not be at the maximum dose, when combination treatment is attempted, in the author's opinion. Adjunctive use of bupropion with clomipramine (Anafranil) should be attempted cautiously, since clomipramine by itself decreases seizure threshold appreciably.

Summary of Advantages and Disadvantages of Bupropion

Advantages

- Effective for atypical depression or mild to moderate depression
- Does not cause sexual dysfunction
- Low anticholinergic side effects
- Low cardiovascular side effects
- Relatively low GI side effects
- Can be used for treatment of ADHD

- Effective for anergia, hypersomnia, apathy, and psychomotor retardation
- Possibly does not increase "cycling" in bipolar depression
- May be occasionally effective in partially restoring sexual function in patients who have sexual dysfunction due to antidepressant treatment
- FDA pregnancy category B

Disadvantages

- Need for strict dose adherence due to seizure risk
- Need for multiple dosing can affect compliance
- Relatively higher incidence of headaches
- Relatively higher incidence of insomnia and anxiety
- Contraindicated in patients with a history of seizure or who are predisposed to seizures or in patients with bulimia/anorexia
- Relatively high cost since several pills are required

A sustained-release (SR) formulation of bupropion is expected to be introduced as 100 and 150 mg dose tablets in December 1996. The SR form has a more convenient BID schedule compared to the currently available immediate release (IR) form which has a TID-QID dosing schedule, making it very inconvenient for most patients to adhere to. Furthermore, the IR form carries a seizure risk slightly higher than that of TCAs. The SR tablet is expected to overcome these problems. BID schedule recommended for the SR form requires a minimum of an eight-hour interval between doses. The maximum single dose for the SR formulation is 200 mg, and maximum daily dose is 200 mg BID (total 400 mg). Compared to the IR form, the SR form provides lower peak bupropion plasma levels and less variability in peak and trough steady-state bupropion plasma concentration. Therefore, the seizure risk of the SR formulation is expected to be lower than that of the IR form of bupropion and might even bring the seizure risk down to the lower levels typically associated with TCAs.

The starting dose may be either 150 mg AM or 100 mg BID. The dose may be increased to 150 mg BID and, if necessary, eventually to 200 mg BID after one to two weeks on a fixed dose. Various dosing regimens are possible within the general dosing guidelines mentioned previously, depending on individual patient needs and characteristics. Some dosing examples are given below.

Bupropion SR dose	Possible clinical applications
100, 150, or 200 mg AM	Elderly, adjunctive use in a combination regimen, mild depression, ADHD, medically ill patients
150 mg BID or 200 mg BID	major depression, dysthymia, ADHD

The dose of the SR form is comparable to the IR form dose except that the maximum recommended SR dose is 200 mg BID (total 400 mg per day), whereas the maximum recommended IR dose is 150 mg TID (total 450 mg per day). The side effects reported for the SR formulation are dry mouth, tremor, sweating, and tinnitus. Based on the experience with IR formulation of bupropion and that of sustained-release formulations of other medications, transient side effects such as headache, nausea, hypermotility of the GI tract, and insomnia (if the second dose is taken close to bedtime) are possibilities. However, widespread clinical use is necessary to completely identify the side effect profile of the SR formulation or any new drug. Combining SR and IR forms is not recommended due to the probability that an IR form could increase the peak plasma bupropion in a patient also taking the SR form, thereby nullifying the improved safety profile of the SR form with regard to seizure risk.

In summary, the SR form is an improvement over the IR form because of decreased seizure risk due to lower peak bupropion plasma levels and a more convenient BID schedule which should result in better patient compliance. The medication cost is expected to be comparable to the IR form.

Summary of Advantages and Disadvantages of Bupropion SR

Advantages

- Effective for depression, particularly if anergia, hypersomnia, apathy, or psychomotor retardation is present
- Can be used for treatment of ADHD
- Does not cause sexual dysfunction
- Low anticholinergic side effects
- Low cardiovascular side effects
- Possibly does not increase cycling in bipolar patients

- May be occasionally effective in partially alleviating antidepressant-induced sexual dysfunction, and possibly effective as an aid to smoking cessation
- FDA pregnancy category B

Disadvantages

- BID dosing, though an improvement over the IR form, can still affect patient compliance to some extent
- At the higher dose range, insomnia, anxiety, and headache can potentially be side effects (These side effects were not frequent in premarketing trials.)
- Seizure risk at 200 mg BID not studied in premarketing trials (Theoretically, the seizure risk of SR formulation is expected to be lower than that of the IR formulation, even at the highest recommended SR dose.)
- Contraindicated in patients with a history of seizures or bulimia/anorexia

FLUOXETINE (PROZAC)

Fluoxetine is a serotonergic antidepressant with antianxiety and anti-obsessive-compulsive effects. It has a half-life of two to three days, and is 95 percent plasma-protein bound. The active metabolite norfluoxetine has a half-life of six to eight days. It is metabolized by the liver and excreted by the kidneys. It is available in 10 mg and 20 mg capsules and in liquid form.

The dosage range is from 10 mg to 80 mg, although most patients respond between 20 mg and 60 mg dose. In rare instances, a dose of 100 mg has been necessary for effectiveness. All of the serotonergic medications are much safer than TCAs in overdose. Fluoxetine is as effective as TCAs, and its side effects are more tolerable than those of TCAs. It has minimal anticholinergic and cardiovascular side effects. The common side effects associated with fluoxetine are nausea, anxiety, insomnia, loss of appetite, sexual dysfunction, mild jaw and neck muscle stiffness, and headaches. Paradoxically, it is used for treatment of intractable headaches. All of the side effects except sexual dysfunction tend to improve over a few weeks. There are fairly successful and simple interventions to deal with all of the common side effects.

Fluoxetine has proven to be particularly effective in patients with anger outbursts, irritability, moodiness, crying spells, excessive emotional sensitivity, obsessive or compulsive characteristics, irrational fears, hypochondriasis, anergia, hypersomnia, anxiety attacks, and hyperphagia. In obsessive-compulsive disorder, the doses tend to be at the higher range, usually 60 mg to 80 mg per day. Fluoxetine is typically started at 20 mg po AM after breakfast because an evening dose interferes with sleep in most patients. Patients should be informed of possible short-term nausea, anxiety, insomnia, heartburn, and sexual dysfunction. They should be assured that, in the majority of patients, most of these side effects subside in seven to ten days. If side effects persist, there are simple and effective medication interventions. In some patients, fluoxetine causes mild sedation and yawning, in which case it may be given at bedtime.

In generalized anxiety disorder, fluoxetine is usually given in low doses, at 5 mg to 20 mg daily. The liquid form is very convenient when an intermediate dose or a dose lower than 10 mg is indicated. Anxiety and an akathisia-like symptom can be initial side effects of fluoxetine for which short-term adjunctive prescription of benzodiazepines may be needed. Fluoxetine can also be effective in patients with hypochondriasis and somatization disorders, which have anxiety and obsessive features as underlying symptoms.

Summary of Advantages and Disadvantages of Fluoxetine

Advantages

- Lack of TCA/MAOI side effects
- Effective for depression, OCD, anxiety, bulimia/anorexia, etc.
- Does not produce weight gain in most patients
- Mild to moderate energizing effects
- Good safety profile for patients with cardiovascular problems
- Long half-life is advantageous should patients forget to take medication occasionally
- Once-a-day administration
- Side effects are usually mild and tend to subside over time
- Tends to cause fewer GI side effects compared to other serotonergic medications
- Safety in overdose

Disadvantages

- Causes insomnia and weight loss in some patients
- Long half-life makes it difficult to switch to other medications, e.g., switching to an MAOI requires five to six weeks wait
- Causes sexual dysfunction (decreased libido, orgasmic and ejaculatory inhibition, or erectile difficulties) in about 60 percent of patients
- High cost of medication due to lack of availability of higher dosage strength; many patients need two to three 20 mg capsules per day, costing $100 to $150 per month
- Initial negative publicity related to a number of unsuccessful lawsuits (both criminal defense and product liability) claiming that fluoxetine induced suicidal and/or homicidal behavior, causing resistance in some patients that is sometimes difficult to overcome despite reassurance (However, lately, the patient resistance has largely subsided and should not be a concern for the prescribing physician.)
- High protein binding causes displacement of other medications with high protein binding, and vice versa (although in most cases, this is not clinically significant)

SERTRALINE (ZOLOFT)

Sertraline is a serotonergic antidepressant that is effective and FDA approved for treatment of depression and obsessive-compulsive disorder. It can also be used for treatment of other conditions, such as anxiety disorder and bulimia/anorexia. Sertraline and its active metabolites have a combined half-life of approximately one to three days. It is about 98 percent protein bound. Sertraline is metabolized by the liver and excreted by the kidneys. It can be given once a day, usually in the morning with breakfast to minimize possible GI irritation and insomnia.

Sertraline has side effects similar to fluoxetine and other SSRIs. However, in the author's experience, it tends to cause nausea and dyspepsia slightly more commonly than fluoxetine, paroxetine, nefazodone, and fluvoxamine. Antacids or H_2 blockers during the first week of sertraline therapy can reduce or prevent GI side effects. Anxiety and insomnia as initial side effects are also seen, but probably less, compared to fluoxetine. Other side effects such as decreased libido and ejaculatory and orgasmic inhibition, insomnia, and slight decrease in appetite are similar to fluoxetine. It should be used with caution in patients taking terfenadine, astemizole, or cisapride due to hepatic enzyme inhibition leading to potential QT prolongation.

It is available in scored tablets in 50 mg and 100 mg strength. The usual dosage range is 50 mg to 200 mg, with the maximum recommended dose being 200 mg. The majority of patients tend to respond optimally at 100 mg, given as a one-time dose in the morning with breakfast to minimize GI side effects and insomnia. Those with generalized anxiety disorder tend to respond at lower dose, such as the 25 mg to 50 mg range, and those with obsessive-compulsive disorder tend to need dosages in the upper ranges such as 200 mg, with most depressions responding in the midrange at 100 mg to 150 mg. Several of the patients who the author had to treat at 300 mg were patients with obsessive-compulsive disorder. Patients who responded at the 300 mg dosage tolerated the medication without significant side effects, except decreased libido and anorgasmia, which can occur at any dosage range.

The cost advantage of sertraline, since it is available in scored tablets at 50 mg and 100 mg dosages, is significant, compared to fluoxetine. The cost of 100 mg pills of sertraline is $60 per month, whereas fairly equivalent doses of fluoxetine at 40 mg (consisting of two 20 mg capsules) will cost about $100 per month, a cost saving of approximately $40 per month at current prices. Those who do well on sertraline 50 mg daily can realize further cost savings by obtaining 100 mg pills and dividing them.

Any medication in tablet form can be similarly divided in individual cases if cost saving can be achieved, except for some of the slow-release preparations in which breaking a tablet can possibly affect the controlled-release function.

Summary of Advantages and Disadvantages of Sertraline

Advantages

- Effective for depression, anxiety, obsessions, compulsions, bulimia, and panic disorder

- Better side effect profile compared to TCAs and MAOIs
- Once-a-day dosing
- Cost advantages as described above
- Flexibility of scored tablet
- Patients with cardiovascular problems are not affected
- Side effects are usually mild and tend to subside over time
- Safety in overdose

Disadvantages

- Slightly higher incidence of nausea and dyspepsia, compared to fluoxetine, but less than venlafaxine (Effexor)
- Sexual dysfunction similar to all other serotonergic medications (approximately 60 percent of patients)
- High protein binding causes displacement of other medications with high protein binding and vice versa (this is not clinically significant in most cases)

PAROXETINE (PAXIL)

Paroxetine is a serotonergic antidepressant with a half-life of 20 hours and 95 percent plasma-protein binding. It is available as tablets in 20 mg scored, and unscored 10 mg, 30 mg, and 40 mg strengths. The dosage range is between 10 mg and 60 mg. Most people respond at 30 mg to 40 mg range. It has no active metabolites. Paroxetine has been found to be effective for the treatment of depression, anxiety disorder, obsessive-compulsive disorder, and bulimia. It is formally approved by the FDA for treatment of depression, obsessive-compulsive disorders, and panic disorder.

Paroxetine can be administered once a day, usually with breakfast to minimize possible GI irritation. It is a more potent serotonin reuptake inhibitor than either fluoxetine or sertraline. In clinical experience, paroxetine tends to have relatively less GI irritation compared to sertraline. The incidence of anxiety as a side effect is less compared to fluoxetine or sertraline. Hence, it is well-suited for patients with anxiety disorder, panic disorders, and obsessive-compulsive disorder, although all serotonergic antidepressants have excellent antianxiety effects. Insomnia as a side effect is also relatively less frequent.

However, relatively greater incidence of sexual side effects such as decreased libido and inhibited orgasm are seen with paroxetine in clinical experience, compared to all other antidepressants, with the possible exception of clomipramine (Anafranil) and MAOIs.

Since paroxetine's half-life is only 20 hours, patients could experience relapse of depression and anxiety, with increased likelihood of withdrawal symptoms such as nausea, GI upset, dizziness, and headaches, if even a few doses are missed. Therefore, the patient should be instructed to remember to take the medication daily. Rarely, patients experience emergence of depression and anxiety symptoms approximately 12 to 16 hours after the morning dose, in which case, half or 1/3 of the morning dose can be administered in the late afternoon which usually controls this problem effectively. When withdrawing from paroxetine, patients should be instructed to taper off by gradually decreasing doses over a period of five to eight days to minimize withdrawal symptoms. If the medication must be stopped abruptly for any reason, reassure the patient that the withdrawal symptoms may be uncomfortable but are not serious. These symptoms generally subside in three to five days. Symptomatic treatment using benzodiazepines or antinausea medications depending on the specific withdrawal symptom may help.

The availability of paroxetine tablets in four different strengths should enable flexible dosing and some cost savings for patients. At a cost of $2 per pill, a patient taking paroxetine 30 mg daily–which is fairly equivalent to 40 mg of fluoxetine (Prozac) and 100 mg of sertraline (Zoloft)–will have to spend approximately $60 per month, making paroxetine comparable to sertraline but less expensive than fluoxetine.

Paroxetine is usually started at 20 mg every morning, preferably after breakfast, with a 10 mg increase every two weeks, up to 60 mg to achieve maximum response. For some patients the dose must be increased to 80 mg (preferably given as one 40 mg dose in the AM and at noon), although 60 mg is the maximum recommended by the drug manufacturer. As with all medications, if intolerable side effects emerge and if they cannot be adequately managed, paroxetine should be discontinued in favor of trying another medication.

Summary of Advantages and Disadvantages of Paroxetine

Advantages

- Effective for depression, anxiety disorders, obsessions, compulsions, eating disorders, and other SSRI indications
- Lack of TCA/MAOI side effects
- No significant weight gain
- No significant GI side effects
- Less incidence of anxiety as a side effect
- Does not commonly cause insomnia
- Safer in overdose, compared to TCAs, bupropion, and MAOIs
- No active metabolites
- Flexible and convenient once-a-day dosing in scored tablet form (the 10 mg, 30 mg, and 40 mg pills are not scored, but can be easily divided)
- Does not have significant cardiovascular side effects
- Fairly short half-life enables switch to other medications more expeditiously
- Clinically significant drug interactions due to hepatic enzyme inhibition or induction are rare

Disadvantages

- Higher incidence of sexual dysfunction, compared to other serotonergic medications (estimated 60 to 70 percent in the author's clinical experience)
- Greater protein binding can displace other drugs that are highly protein bound (although not clinically significant in most cases)
- Short half-life tends to lead to rapid reemergence of depressive/anxiety symptoms and/or emergence of withdrawal symptoms if patient misses medication for several days or abruptly stops taking medication

VENLAFAXINE (EFFEXOR)

The antidepressant venlafaxine is a serotonin and norepinephrine reuptake inhibitor with a half-life of approximately five hours and plasma protein binding of about 28 percent. It is available as scored tablets in quite a range of doses at 25, 37.5, 50, 75, and 100 mg. Its serotonergic and norepinephrinergic actions make it truly a "broad-spectrum" antidepressant much like imipramine. In clinical practice, venlafaxine appears to be as effective as imipramine, other TCAs, and MAOIs in the treatment of depression. However, the significant advantage of venlafaxine, compared to TCAs and MAOIs, is the lack of TCA side effects. It tends to cause mild elevation in blood pressure; hence, regular blood pressure monitoring in those who have hypertension or borderline hypertension, especially in the initial three to four weeks of beginning treatment and after each dose increase, is strongly recommended.

The effective dosage range is between 75 mg and 300 mg in two or three divided doses. The maximum recommended dose is 375 mg per day in divided doses. Venlafaxine weakly inhibits reuptake of dopamine at the higher dosage range, although the clinical significance of this phenomenon is not clear. The author has no experience in treating patients at higher than the maximum dosage of 375 mg per day in divided doses.

The theoretical advantage of venlafaxine is its broad-spectrum activity and hence its likelihood to treat depression that is mediated by serotonin as well as norepinephrine. There is a claim that venlafaxine tends to energize patients due to its activity on the norepinephrine neurotransmitter system. From the author's clinical experience in treating in excess of 100 patients on venlafaxine, some of them at 375 mg a day, the energizing effects are comparable to other energizing serotonergic medications such as fluoxetine and sertraline. In this respect, theoretical expectation and clinical experience correlate only to a limited extent. The incidence of nausea and dyspepsia seems to be slightly higher compared to other serotonergic antidepressants, with the incidence of sexual side effects similar to other SSRIs. Prophylactic administration of antacids or H_2 blockers during the first week of venlafaxine therapy could reduce the incidence of GI side effects.

The scored-tablet and multiple-strength formats allow flexible dosing, enabling some cost advantages for the patient especially at the lower dosage range, where a 100 mg strength tablet at a cost of approximately $1.25 can be divided for twice-a-day dosing. Venlafaxine at a dose of 200 mg per day will cost approximately $57 per month, as compared to a fairly equivalent dose of fluoxetine at 40 mg per day costing $100 per month, sertraline at 100 mg daily costing approximately $60 per month, and paroxetine at 30 mg daily costing approximately $60 per month, making venlafaxine one of the least expensive of the new generation of antidepressants. Since most patients respond at 150 mg per day or less, and since scored tablets up to 100 mg strength are available, the cost saving is even greater.

Venlafaxine is usually started at 25 mg three times a day with meals to minimize GI side effects. This can be prescribed as 25 mg po TID, or 50 mg 1/2 tablet po TID. Higher starting doses increase the chance of gastrointestinal side effects. Further dose increases at a rate of 75 mg per week may be attempted every week, until satisfactory clinical response is seen or side effects interfere with treatment, up to the maximum dose of 375 mg per day in divided doses.

Since venlafaxine tends to work somewhat faster, if no improvement is found on a steady dose in a week, a further dose increase of 50 to 75 mg per week may be attempted. There are a few patients who may respond at very low doses such as 25 mg to 50 mg taken as a one-time dose. Venlafaxine does not frequently cause insomnia and in a fair number of cases, has been found to improve sleep, making a bedtime dose appropriate. Since venlafaxine binds protein only at 28 percent, it does not alter the serum levels of other drugs that are highly protein bound; this is an advantage compared to other serotonergic drugs, all of which are highly protein bound.

Since venlafaxine has a short half-life, multiple dosing is needed. This characteristic increases the chances of emergence of withdrawal symptoms on abrupt discontinuation of the medication. Gradual tapering over five to seven days is recommended. Greater patient motivation is required for compliance with multiple dosing schedules.

Summary of Advantages and Disadvantages of Venlafaxine

Advantages

- Broad spectrum of activity
- Effective in treatment of depression, atypical depression, anxiety disorders, obsessive-compulsive disorder, bulimia, etc.
- Low protein binding, offering increased safety in use with patients on medications that are highly bound to plasma protein

– Possible faster onset of action
– Cost advantages and dosing flexibility; at low dosage ranges, venlafaxine is the least expensive of the serotonergic antidepressants, making it the "best buy" in the author's cost comparison
– Lack of TCA/MAOI side effects
– No significant weight gain
– No active metabolites
– Safer in overdose, compared to TCA/MAOI or bupropion
– Short half-life enables faster switch to other medications such as MAOIs
– Clinically significant drug interactions due to hepatic enzyme inhibition or induction are rare

Disadvantages

– Nausea and dyspepsia are common initial side effects
– Tendency to cause mild increase in blood pressure in some patients
– Need for multiple dosing requires greater patient motivation
– Short half-life can lead to reemergence of depression/anxiety symptoms or emergence of withdrawal symptoms if several doses are missed or medication is abruptly discontinued
– Sexual side effects similar to other SSRIs

FLUVOXAMINE (LUVOX)

Fluvoxamine is a serotonergic antidepressant approved for treatment of obsessive-compulsive disorder, with a half-life of 16 hours and protein binding at 80 percent. It may also be used for treatment of depression, anxiety disorders, and eating disorders. Fluvoxamine is available in scored tablets in 50 mg and 100 mg strengths. It is contraindicated in patients taking terfenadine (Seldane), cisapride (Propulsid), or astemizole (Hismanal), due to rare risk of cardiac arrhythmia resulting from QT prolongation.

Fluvoxamine has all of the advantages of serotonergic antidepressants, with a similar side effect profile; however, there are some differences that are clinically important. Since insomnia is not a common side effect, it may be started in the evening or at bedtime as a once-a-day 50 mg or 100 mg dose. Anxiety as a side effect is relatively less frequent than with other serotonergic antidepressants; GI side effects are similar to other SSRIs. Sexual dysfunction tends to be somewhat less compared to other SSRIs, estimated at 40 percent in the author's clinical experience. It has been effective in the treatment of obsessive-compulsive disorder in some patients who did not respond satisfactorily to clomipramine (Anafranil), fluoxetine (Prozac), or other SSRIs, suggesting that it is a useful option among SSRIs for treatment of obsessive-compulsive disorder. Hence, overall efficacy is estimated to be similar to fluoxetine, sertraline and paroxetine for treatment of obsessive-compulsive disorder. The maximum dose recommended is 300 mg per day, in divided dosages. It is started at 50 mg or 100 mg at bedtime, with a 50 mg increase as needed every two weeks until the maximum dose of 300 mg is reached. The average effective dose is 100 to 200 mg per day. The availability of the scored-tablet form in 50 mg and 100 mg strengths offers flexibility of dosing and possible cost savings especially at lower doses. For example, it will cost a patient approximately $85 per month on fluvoxamine 150 mg daily, compared to sertraline (Zoloft) 100 mg daily costing $60 per month, fluoxetine (Prozac) 40 mg costing $100 per month, paroxetine (Paxil) 30 mg costing $60 per month, and venlafaxine (Effexor) 100 mg costing $40 per month.

Summary of Advantages and Disadvantages of Fluvoxamine

Advantages

- Effective for treatment of obsessive-compulsive disorder (the only FDA approved use in the United States at present), depression, anxiety disorders, and bulimia
- Lack of TCA side effects
- Fairly safe in overdose (as with all SSRIs)
- Comparatively low incidence of sexual dysfunction (estimated at 40 percent, which is still significant, but lower than other SSRIs)
- Flexible dosing and possible cost saving, due to scored-tablet form in 50 mg and 100 mg strengths
- Low incidence of insomnia, anxiety, and weight gain as side effects

–No active metabolites
–Does not have significant cardiovascular side effects
–Once-a-day bedtime dosing convenient for most patients

Disadvantages

–Causes GI side effects similar to most SSRIs
–Current FDA approval only for obsessive-compulsive disorder (although this does not prevent physicians from using it for other conditions such as depression, anxiety, bulimia, etc.)

NEFAZODONE (SERZONE)

Nefazodone is an antidepressant with several actions at the synapse. It is an inhibitor of serotonin reuptake, and a serotonin receptor blocker. To a lesser extent, it inhibits norepinephrine reuptake. Thus, it shares some of the neurotransmitter dynamics of trazodone (Desyrel) and venlafaxine (Effexor). Although nefazodone is formally approved by the FDA for treatment of depression, it has broader clinical applications as do all antidepressants; for example, in treatment of anxiety, phobic and obsessive-compulsive disorders, post-traumatic stress disorder, etc. It tends to cause sexual dysfunction less frequently compared to SSRIs. As with other SSRIs, it is devoid of anticholinergic side effects, and has very low cardiovascular toxicity. Nefazodone potentiates the effects of alprazolam (Xanax) and triazolam (Halcion) by increasing their blood levels; hence, the dosage of the latter two medications should by reduced by 1/2 to 1/3 if nefazodone is added. The hepatic metabolism of terfenadine (Seldane), astemizole (Hismanal), and cisapride (Propulsid) can be inhibited by nefazodone, leading to potential toxicity and prolongation of QT interval. Therefore nefazodone is contraindicated with these drugs. Loratadine (Claritin) does not cause significant interaction with nefazodone.

It has a half-life of approximately six hours and is highly plasma-protein bound. Available dosages are 100, 150, 200, and 250 mg tablets. Typical effective dosage range is between 300 mg and 500 mg in divided doses, the major portion preferably given at bedtime. The maximum dose is 600 mg per day. A dose of 300 mg or less may be given in one bedtime dose if daytime sedation or insomnia is a problem.

Clinical experience based on prescribing nefazodone to both inpatients and outpatients has revealed that its effectiveness in treating severe depression and anxiety is comparable to a range between that of SSRIs and trazodone. Its mildly sedating property and relatively low interference with sexual functioning as seen in clinical practice so far are clear advantages over SSRIs and MAOIs, particularly for treating mild to moderate depression. The estimate of sexual dysfunction associated with nefazodone is at 15 percent in the author's clinical experience, compared to 60 percent associated with SSRIs. When sexual dysfunction occurs with nefazodone, the severity is also less. The most frequently reported side effects of nefazodone are somnolence, nausea, dizziness, asthenia, lightheadedness, dry mouth, constipation, blurred vision, and confusion. Postural hypotension can occur in susceptible patients, such as patients with cardiovascular or cerebrovascular disease, or patients taking antihypertensive medication. Most of the side effects subside during the first one to two weeks of nefazodone therapy. Since nefazodone is fairly new, additional clinical experience will further clarify nefazodone's therapeutic and side effect profile in relation to established antidepressants.

The cost for a patient on nefazodone 200 mg twice a day for one month is approximately $40, compared to fluvoxamine (Luvox) 150 mg daily costing $85 per month, venlafaxine (Effexor) 100 mg twice a day costing $57 per month, paroxetine (Paxil) 30 mg daily costing $60 per month, sertraline (Zoloft) 100 mg daily costing $60 per month, and fluoxetine (Prozac) 40 mg daily costing $100 per month. Nefazodone offers significant cost advantages compared to SSRIs and bupropion, as evident from this comparative cost analysis.

Although the manufacturer's recommendation is to start patients at 100 mg twice a day, given the frequent complaint of nausea, the author's suggestion is to start nefazodone at 50 mg three times a day with meals to minimize GI side effects, in spite of the slight decrease in bioavailability when taken with food. After about five days, the dose may be doubled to 100 mg three times a day with meals. After the patient is tolerant of the possible GI side effects, the dosing schedule may be changed to twice a day, with the major dose given at bedtime. Dosage increases over 300 mg are usually achieved at a rate of 100 mg increment per week, up to a maximum of 600 mg per day in two to three divided doses, unless side effects interfere. For the elderly and medically ill, dosage should be reduced by half.

Summary of Advantages and Disadvantages of Nefazodone

Advantages

- Effective for treatment of mild to moderate depression and anxiety
- Lack of TCA side effects
- Significantly less incidence of sexual dysfunction, compared to SSRIs
- Safety profile similar to SSRIs
- Relatively low cost (a "best buy")
- May aid sleep when given at bedtime
- Low incidence of weight gain

Disadvantages

- Nausea, sedation, and dizziness can be initial side effects
- Need for multiple-dosing schedule
- High protein binding causes displacement of other drugs that are protein bound (although this is not clinically significant in most cases)
- Antidepressant efficacy is only modest for treatment of severe depression, compared to that of SSRIs, TCAs, and MAOIs (but superior to that of trazodone in the author's clinical experience so far)

MIRTAZAPINE (REMERON)

Mirtazapine is an antidepressant with noradrenergic and serotonergic pharmacological actions, introducted in the United States in August 1996. Its presynaptic α_2 (Alpha-2) adrenoreceptor antagonism stimulates release of norepinephrine and serotonin. It has a half-life of approximately 30 hours, making it suitable for once-a-day dosing. Plasma-protein binding is estimated at 85 percent. It is eliminated by hepatic metabolism and excreted by the kidneys; therefore, dosage adjustment may be necessary for the hepatically and renally impaired. Mirtazapine is available in scored 15 mg and 30 mg tablets. The effective dosage range recommended by the manufacturer is 15 to 45 mg, preferably given at bedtime.

The side effect profile of mirtazapine is different from that of SSRIs and TCAs. Common side effects include sedation, increased appetite, weight gain, dizziness, orthostatic hypotension, malaise, apathy, anxiety, and agitation. Most patients eventually develop tolerance to the side effects. In premarketing clinical trials, two out of 2,796 patients exposed to mirtazapine developed agranulocytosis, and a third patient developed severe neutropenia, yielding a crude incidence of severe neutropenia of 1 per 1,000 patients. Mirtazapine should be discontinued if signs of infection such as flu-like symptoms, sore throat, fever, chills, fatigue, or stomatitis develop along with a low WBC count. Although the incidence of agranulocytosis associated with mirtazapine is extremely low, it is relatively contraindicated with clozapine because of potential for additive risk of suppression of bone marrow. WBC monitoring is not routinely recommended for patients taking mirtazapine.

Mirtazapine does not cause significant sexual dysfunction. Its sedative effects could be exploited in patients who have insomnia by giving the dosage at bedtime. However, the author's limited clinical experience with mirtazapine so far has indicated that approximately 50 percent of patients had difficulty tolerating mirtazapine due to daytime sedation, a "drugged" feeling, activation at nighttime, and restlessness when the medication was started with the first dose at 15 mg daily, as suggested by the drug manufacturer. Hence the author's current practice is to start mirtazapine at 3.75 mg (1/4 tablet) or 7.5 mg (1/2 tablet) at HS for the first four days before gradually increasing the dose. Since antidepressants may take from two to four weeks for response, it is prudent to wait a minimum of two weeks in an outpatient setting prior to increasing the dose beyond 15 mg daily, which is considered a low therapeutic dose. In partial responders, addition of a low dose of an SSRI such as fluoxetine 10 to 20 mg, paroxetine 10 to 20 mg, or sertraline 25 to 50 mg in AM may be effective in some patients. If activation is predominant in a particular patient, mirtazapine may be switched to AM schedule. A 14-day drug washout interval is required between administration of mirtazapine and MAOIs. Additional clinical experience will provide more definitive information as to the drug's effectiveness, tolerability, and patient acceptance in an outpatient practice environment. The price of mirtazapine 30 pills (15 mg or 30 mg) is approximately $60, which compares favorably with the price of SSRIs.

Summary of Advantages and Disadvantages of Mirtazapine (Remeron)

Advantages

- Effective for depression; possibly effective for anxiety at a low dose
- Once-a-day dosing
- Lack of sexual dysfunction
- Flexibility of a scored tablet
- Safer than TCAs in overdose
- Not a significant inhibitor of cytochrome P450 enzymes
- Does not affect cardiac conduction at therapeutic doses

Disadvantages

- Sedation, somnolence, dizziness and activation excessive unless starting dose is 7.5 mg or less; tolerance to side ffects may take several weeks*
- Patient tolerance is somewhat less compared to SSRIs; tolerance is comparable to TCAs (secondary amines); better tolerated than tertiary amines*

*These observations are primarily based on the author's limited clinical experience of treating approximately 40 patients using mirtazapine at the time of this writing.

– Rare incidence of agranulocytosis (estimated at 1.1 per 1,000 patients); need to warn patients of this risk and to report signs of infection; can affect patient acceptance

CLOMIPRAMINE (ANAFRANIL)

Clomipramine is a tricyclic antidepressant approved and primarily used for treatment of obsessive-compulsive disorder. It has relatively more potent serotonergic effects compared to its norepinephrinergic properties. Although its FDA approval is for treatment of obsessive-compulsive disorder, it can be used as an antidepressant and an antianxiety medication, as can all TCAs. It has a half-life of 30 hours, and is 95 percent protein bound. Clomipramine is available in 25, 50, and 75 mg capsules. Treatment is started at 25 mg BID with 25 mg increments every two to three days until a dose of 150 mg is reached. Thereafter, dosage is increased by 25 mg per week if needed, up to a maximum dose of 250 mg per day in divided doses.

Clomipramine, being a tricyclic antidepressant, has significant anticholinergic and other typical tricyclic side effects. In addition, it tends to lower seizure threshold more than other antidepressants. Hence, the maximum recommended dose of 250 mg per day should not be exceeded. While all antidepressants except perhaps MAOIs and SSRIs lower seizure threshold, in the author's experience the incidence of generalized seizures precipitated by clomipramine is higher than any antidepressant including bupropion (Wellbutrin) at comparable dosage range. Therefore, the author has a conservative approach of not exceeding clomipramine 225 mg per day and not exceeding 150 mg per dose to keep the seizure risk low. As in the case of bupropion, patients on clomipramine should be educated about the increased seizure risk and strictly cautioned not to exceed dosage limits. If a patient who is at increased risk for seizures for any reason needs to be on clomipramine, prophylactic anticonvulsant treatment should be considered while the patient is on clomipramine. The caution regarding slightly increased seizure risk is given by the author only in cases where the dosage exceeds 150 mg per day; the clinician must maintain a balance between encouraging and reassuring the patient and frightening the patient by listing side effects that are rare and hence of no practical significance. The common side effects of clomipramine are dose-dependent in a fairly linear fashion. They are dry mouth, blurry vision, constipation, increased heart rate, sedation, weight gain, and increased sweating. Most of these side effects subside over a period of two to three weeks, although sweating and sedation often persist. TCAs can exacerbate narrow-angle glaucoma. The patient can also develop postural hypotension and slowing of cardiac conduction. Central nervous system side effects include sedation, lethargy, and a central anticholinergic syndrome, particularly in elderly patients on high doses. Sexual dysfunction such as decreased libido, erectile difficulties and inhibited orgasm are also fairly common, estimated at 60 to 70 percent. Sexual dysfunction associated with clomipramine is higher than with other TCAs.

Summary of Advantages and Disadvantages of Clomipramine

Advantages

- The most effective medication for obsessive-compulsive disorder
- Effective for depression and anxiety
- Less weight gain, compared to other TCAs

Disadvantages

- Lethal in overdose
- Significantly lowers seizure threshold at high doses
- Moderate anticholinergic side effects
- Affects cardiac conduction at high doses
- Greater risk of interaction with over-the-counter medications and alcohol (as compared with new generation antidepressants)
- Poorly tolerated by the elderly and medically ill, at high doses

NALTREXONE (REVIA, TREXAN)

Naltrexone is an opioid antagonist, approved for use in the treatment of alcoholism. Naltrexone at 50 mg daily decreases the relapse rates in alcoholics when used in conjunction with psychosocial and group therapy approaches (such as Alcoholics Anonymous). It controls relapse by decreasing cravings for alcohol and, to some extent, by inhibiting the hedonistic effects of alcohol. The author's experience in treating a number of patients on naltrexone supports the expectations described above. Naltrexone may be effective as an adjunctive medication in controlling the compulsive self-mutilation behavior frequently associated with borderline personality disorder. It is available as a 50 mg tablet. Although its half-life is only about four hours, its antialcohol effects last longer, enabling once a day administration.

Side effects include anxiety, depression, nausea, and anergia during the first several months of treatment. It can cause an elevation of liver enzymes requiring periodic tests to monitor liver function. Administration of naltrexone to patients on opioids can precipitate sudden opioid withdrawal. Patients should be free of opioids for at least seven days before starting naltrexone.

Since many alcoholics have hepatic dysfunction, baseline liver function tests and biweekly monitoring of liver enzymes are prudent during the first two months of treatment, with a decreased frequency of laboratory monitoring thereafter. Naltrexone costs approximately $150 for 30 pills. If price is not a deterrent, its use should be encouraged in patients with alcohol dependence because of its beneficial effects.

Chapter 15

Clinical Profiles of Selected New Generation Antipsychotics

RISPERIDONE (RISPERDAL)

Risperidone is a serotonin-dopamine receptor antagonist, approved for the treatment of psychotic disorders. It is metabolized by the cytochrome P-450 enzyme system and has an active metabolite. Its half-life is 20 hours and plasma protein binding is 90 percent. Its metabolism can be inhibited by drugs that inhibit cytochrome P-450 II D6, such as fluoxetine, paroxetine, sertraline, and quinidine. It can interfere with, or its metabolism can be interfered by, other drugs that are metabolized by the cytochrome P-450 II D6 enzyme. Examples of such drugs include nortriptyline, desipramine, fluoxetine, paroxetine, beta-blockers, and various antipsychotics. A slight dosage reduction of risperidone should be considered if any of the above medications are coadministered. As with almost all medications, the dosage should be decreased in elderly patients and in patients who have liver disease or renal impairment. Its alpha-adrenergic blocking effect can cause orthostatic hypotension, tachycardia, dizziness, and syncope in patients susceptible to hypotension and in patients with cardiovascular disease. Lower initial dosage and slower increments are recommended in these patients.

The significant advantage of risperidone compared to traditional antipsychotics is that it has a low incidence of extrapyramidal symptoms in the optimal therapeutic dose range of 2 to 6 mg daily, and is believed to have a decreased risk of inducing tardive dyskinesia, although many more years of clinical experience will be necessary to obtain any conclusive information regarding the tardive dyskinesia risk. Risk of acute dystonia and neuroleptic malignant syndrome

(NMS) is present but may be lower in comparison to traditional high-potency antipsychotics. The risk of EPS rises in a dose-dependent manner above a dose of 4 to 6 mg daily. Clinical experience so far has confirmed the expectation of lower extrapyramidal symptoms. The possibility (and probability) of decreased risk of tardive dyskinesia should make risperidone attractive to psychiatrists and other physicians treating patients on an antipsychotic. The only other antipsychotics currently available in the United States with decreased risk of tardive dyskinesia, low extrapyramidal symptoms, and effectiveness for negative and positive symptoms are olanzapine (Zyprexa) and clozapine (Clozaril). However, clozapine has a 1 percent risk of lethal agranulocytosis (and 3 to 5 percent risk of seizures in therapeutic doses), requiring mandatory weekly WBC (white blood cell count) for as long as the patient is on the medication. Risperidone and olanzapine have no such risks, avoiding the need for laboratory monitoring. Although clozapine is superior to risperidone in terms of a fairly balanced effectiveness for positive and negative symptoms, clozapine's potential for serious side effects and consequent need for weekly WBC monitoring make it a complicated medication. Hence clozapine's FDA approved use is reserved for treatment of refractory cases of schizophrenia in current clinical practice. Risperidone is effective in treating positive symptoms, such as hallucinations, delusions, agitation, hostility, anxiety, ideas of reference, thought disorders, pressured speech, etc., and fairly effective for improving negative or "deficit" symptoms, such as apathy, social withdrawal, ambivalence, dysphoria, anergia, demoralization, lack of spontaneity, poor initiative, constricted or blunted affect, and concrete thinking.

For treatment of psychotic symptoms that are less acute or those that are likely to be fairly transient, the risperidone dosage range can be from 0.5 mg to 2 mg per day. Many patients with mild psychotic symptoms do well on a dose of risperidone 0.5 mg daily. For the above indications, the length of treatment is usually several weeks to several months, after which the dose is gradually tapered off over a period of several weeks.

Risperidone can cause insomnia in some patients. In these cases, AM administration is preferred. Most patients are able to tolerate dosage at bedtime. The most common side effects include extrapyramidal symptoms, insomnia, fatigue, anxiety, somnolence, hyperprolactinemia, and galactorrhea.

For patients with acute and chronic psychotic conditions, the starting dose recommended by the author is 0.5 mg po QID for two days, increased by 1 milligram increments every two days until 4 mg per day is reached. The 4 mg dose should be maintained for one week before further dosage increase is considered, because clinical experience suggests that most patients respond well at 4 mg or less per day. For the elderly, debilitated, hypotensive, and renally or hepatically impaired patients, the initial dose should be 0.5 mg per day or 0.5 mg BID, with a dosage increase of 0.5 mg per day every two to three days until 2 mg per day is reached. These patients should be kept on 2 mg per day in divided doses for a week prior to considering dosage adjustment.

Risperidone may be combined with antidepressants, anticholinergics, anxiolytics, and mood stabilizers. Occasionally it is combined with clozapine, chlorpromazine, and thioridazine for optimal clinical response including sedation.

Risperidone is available in liquid and tablet form for oral use in doses of 1, 2, 3, and 4 mg strengths. The tablet can be easily broken into smaller doses. Given the high cost of risperidone, it makes sense to obtain the higher dose tablet and divide it. For example, if a patient is on 1 mg per day, there may be some savings by purchasing seven 4 mg tablets and dividing each pill into four, yielding a four week supply (see Table 15.1). Once the patient is stabilized on a dose, minor variations in dose that may occur when a pill is

TABLE 15.1. Costs for Daily Dosage of Risperidone

Daily Risperidone Dose	Quantity	Cost per Month	Cost per Pill	Cost per 1 mg Unit
1 mg	30	$ 60	$2.00	$2.00
2 mg	30	$ 95	$3.16	$1.58
3 mg	30	$120	$4.00	$1.33
4 mg	30	$158	$5.26	$1.31

divided into smaller pieces is not likely to be clinically significant, particularly since risperidone has a half-life of 20 hours.

Summary of Advantages and Disadvantages of Risperidone

Advantages

- Superior effectiveness for positive symptoms of psychosis
- Moderately effective for negative symptoms
- Fairly low incidence of extrapyramidal symptoms and neuroleptic malignant syndrome, compared to traditional high-potency antipsychotics (dose-dependent)
- Mild antianxiety and antidepressant effects at low doses
- Well tolerated by most patients
- First-line general purpose antipsychotic for a broad range of psychotic conditions and for all severity levels; effective for first-episode psychosis and some treatment-resistant schizophrenics
- Possible decreased risk of tardive dyskinesia, compared to traditional antipsychotics (many more years of experience will be necessary to obtain actual estimates)
- Availability of liquid form
- Improved efficacy and tolerability decreases relapses and hospitalizations
- Potential significant long-term cost savings due to decreased illness-related direct and indirect costs

Disadvantages

- Risk of tardive dyskinesia, although considered less frequent than that of traditional antipsychotics, is still present
- Can cause extrapyramidal symptoms and neuroleptic malignant syndrome at the higher dosage range of 6 to 18 mg daily
- High cost of medication (average cost of $2,100 per year for a patient on a dose of 2 mg BID)
- Parenteral form not available, as of this writing
- Increases prolactin level, as do all of the traditional antipsychotics

CLOZAPINE (CLOZARIL)

In terms of overall efficacy for improvement in both positive and negative symptoms, clozapine is clearly superior to all antipsychotics currently available in the United States, including risperidone and olanzapine. Clozapine has a half-life of 12 hours and is 95 percent bound to plasma protein. It is available in 25 mg and 100 mg tablets. Clozapine is approved by the FDA for use in patients with treatment-resistant schizophrenia who fail to respond satisfactorily to at least two standard antipsychotic medications. Weekly monitoring of the WBC is required for the duration of treatment and for four weeks after it is discontinued. Because of the rare incidence of syncope, respiratory depression, and respiratory collapse, the starting dose should be 12.5 mg once or twice the first day, preferably after safely discontinuing benzodiazepines, which tend to increase the chances of respiratory depression–a concern primarily in the elderly. If the patient tolerates the first day's dose well, the dosage may be increased by 25 to 50 mg daily, up to 450 mg over a period of two weeks. If further dosage increase is necessary, it is implemented by maximum increments of 100 mg per week up to a maximum dose of 900 mg per day. Clinical experience indicates that most patients respond satisfactorily to between 200 and 500 mg per day in divided doses. The initial clozapine dosage titration schedule recommended by Sandoz Pharmaceuticals is listed in Table 15.2. Some elderly patients may require a lower startup dose of 6.25 mg and slower titration.

Since clozapine is highly protein-bound, it can displace other highly protein-bound drugs and increase their levels. This is of concern primarily for drugs that have a relatively narrow therapeutic range, for example warfarin or digoxin, though the possible increase in the free-drug level in plasma of these latter medications is considered temporary because of compensatory hepatic clearance.

Clozapine has been used successfully in the treatment of schizoaffective disorder when the patient is not responding well to a combination of traditional antipsychotics, antidepressants, and/or mood stabilizers. It has also been successful in the treatment of complicated and chronic rapid-cycling bipolar disorder, which is unresponsive to standard combination treatment, particularly if antipsychotics in moderate to high doses are required to control the symptoms and to maintain stability. In any psychotic disorder of a chronic nature requiring at least moderate doses of antipsychotics, clozapine could be considered as an option, particularly if traditional antipsychotics are not fully effective. As is true with all antipsychotics, clozapine has

TABLE 15.2. Sandoz-Recommended Initial Clozapine Dosage Titration Schedule

Week 1	AM (mg)	HS (mg)	Total (mg)
Day 1	12.5	12.5*	12.5 - 25
Day 2	25	----	25
Day 3	25	25	50
Day 4	25	50	75
Day 5	50	50	100
Day 6	50	75	125
Day 7	50	100	150
Week 2	**AM (mg)**	**HS (mg)**	**Total (mg)**
Day 8	50	100	150
Day 9	100	100	200
Day 10	100	100	200
Day 11	50	200	250
Day 12	50	200	250
Day 13	100	200	300
Day 14	100	200	300

*Optional

antimanic properties. Moreover, it seems to have mood-stabilizing properties, unlike traditional antipsychotics. Given its risk of agranulocytosis and seizures, clozapine should not be used as a first-line drug for bipolar disorders. However, for treatment-resistant and chronic bipolar patients who do not respond well to antidepressants, traditional antipsychotics, mood stabilizers, and ECT or combinations, clozapine should be considered. For chronic conditions that have a high risk of suicide, such as severe depression with psychotic features, severe dysphoric mania, severe rapid-cycling bipolar disorder, or severe borderline personality disorder with regressive and dissociative features, or any other severe chronic conditions with regressive or psychotic features, a trial of clozapine with its 1 percent risk of agranulocytosis and 3 to 5 percent risk of seizures is a risk worth taking for the patient if other antipsychotics have given suboptimal results since clozapine leads to significant clinical improvement. Similarly, if a patient has extreme homicidal hostility that is chronic and is unresponsive to all other medications, a clozapine trial should be considered. The severe chronic obsessive-compulsive disorder patient with regressive characteristics, psychotic features, and significant functional deterioration, intractable to aggressive standard treatment attempts, is a clinically justifiable candidate for a clozapine trial (prior to considering cingulotomy). In all of these cases, benefit-to-risk ratio related to the use of clozapine is favorable, in the author's opinion.

Clozapine may be considered for treatment of various chronic and severe treatment-refractory and dysfunctional conditions which would benefit from long-term maintenance on an antipsychotic, as listed below.

- Treatment refractory schizophrenia (the only FDA-approved indication)
- All schizophrenias
- Schizoaffective disorders
- Treatment-refractory delusional disorders with severe dysfunction
- All chronic psychotic disorders
- Treatment-refractory severe bipolar disorders with predominant manic and/or psychotic features
- Treatment-refractory severe obsessive compulsive disorder, prior to considering cingulotomy
- Treatment-refractory severe borderline personality disorder, with psychotic and dissociative features
- Treatment-refractory severe depression with psychotic features
- Treatment-refractory severe impulse control disorders
- Treatment-refractory severe dissociative disorders
- Treatment-emergent tardive dyskinesia/tardive dystonia
- Psychotic patients with idiopathic parkinsonism who poorly tolerate other antipsychotics
- Psychosis induced by dopaminergic antiparkinsonian medications

Schizophrenia by definition is a chronic condition. If the diagnosis of schizophrenia can be confirmed, especially if the subtype is that of the disorganized or undifferentiated type with young age at onset (in which the course is expected to be very chronic and where the prognosis is poor), it is the author's opinion that clozapine should be offered to the patient as a first-line maintenance medication. This eliminates the likelihood that the patient and family will go through the agony of multiple antipsychotic medication failures. Although risperidone is a significant improvement over the traditional antipsychotics, clozapine is clearly more effective for negative symptoms compared to risperidone, and hence has overall superiority in the treatment of poor prognosis types of schizophrenia. Additionally, it has been the author's experience that insight, judgment, compliance, and acceptance of the chronic nature of the illness and recognition of the need for continuing on the medication are improved once the patient achieves stabilization on clozapine. As a result, a great majority of patients comply with weekly monitoring of the WBC. This is somewhat surprising, given a history of noncompliance with traditional antipsychotics among such patients, despite requiring weekly needle sticks which is not a pleasant experience.

The combination of clozapine with other medications such as valproate, lithium, antidepressants, benzodiazepines, and low doses of high-potency neuroleptics including risperidone has been successfully used by the author.

At a clozapine dosage in the range of 400 mg to 600 mg per day, the incidence of seizures is estimated at 5 percent, which is a substantial risk. Therefore, the author routinely prescribes prophylactic valproate if clozapine dosage exceeds 500 mg per day. When this combination is used, liver function tests should be monitored to detect any additive liver toxicity. Gabapentin (Neurontin) and lamotrigine (Lamictal) are options if valproate is not tolerated or is ineffective.

Clozapine can be combined with lithium, but must be monitored closely for increased central nervous system side effects. Many patients on clozapine will benefit from adjunctive treatment using serotonergic antidepressants, which have the potential to further improve negative symptoms, especially dysphoria, obsessive worrying, anxiety, demoralization, apathy, and anergia. Fluoxetine and paroxetine can increase clozapine level slightly by inhibition of cytochrome P-450 II D6. Venlafaxine, sertraline, fluvoxamine, and nefazodone do not affect clozapine metabolism significantly. Liver enzyme inhibition should be a clinical consideration only if the patient is already on a high dose of clozapine, or if the dose of the antidepressant is at or near the maximum dosage limit.

Clozapine can be successfully employed in the treatment of patients with parkinsonism accompanied by psychotic symptoms. The dosage in this population is usually on the low range, for example between 25 mg and 100 mg per day.

Unlike traditional antipsychotics and risperidone, clozapine does not affect libido or sexual functioning significantly. Since clozapine has sedative properties, no additional sleep medication is necessary in most cases.

If clinical improvement is noted below the dose of 600 mg per day, there is probably no need for a clozapine blood level. Levels are recommended (1) if toxicity is suspected, (2) to monitor compliance if there is a question regarding this, (3) to guide dosage at the higher dosage range with its increased risks of side effects, (4) if other medications that inhibit clozapine's hepatic metabolism are concurrently used, and (5) to guide dosage adjustment in nonresponders. It is not necessary to obtain clozapine blood levels routinely. A plasma clozapine concentration above 350 ng/mL, or a total plasma concentration of clozapine plus the active metabolite norclozapine above 450 ng/mL is correlated with a high probability of response. The upper therapeutic range of plasma clozapine levels and toxic levels have not been determined. The author has patients who responded satisfactorily at a blood level of less than 200 ng/mL, and at a blood level above 900 ng/mL (without toxic effects).

Clozapine is contraindicated in patients with myeloproliferative disorders. If patients with a low seizure threshold need clozapine, prophylactic treatment with an anticonvulsant should be considered even at low doses of clozapine. Seizure disorder is not a contraindication to the use of clozapine if the seizure is well-controlled on an antiseizure medication and if clozapine is initiated slowly and cautiously with close monitoring of seizure status. Carbamazepine should be avoided in a patient on clozapine because of carbamazepine's potential effects on bone marrow. Cigarette smoking and phenytoin (Dilantin) can decrease clozapine blood levels, and cimetidine (Tagamet) can increase blood levels. Hence, smoking should be discouraged, and the clozapine dose may need adjustment if these medications are started or stopped in a patient on clozapine.

Since the greatest risk of agranulocytosis is within the first six months of starting clozapine, it is reasonable to decrease the frequency of CBC monitoring to biweekly or monthly intervals after the first six months to one year. However, weekly monitoring of the WBC is required currently for as long as the patient is on clozapine, and for four weeks after stopping clozapine. Patients should be instructed to call the physician if any signs of infection are noted such as fever, sore throat, pallor, tonsillitis, flu, pneumonia, lethargy, urinary symptoms, etc. Such precautions could alert the patient to any precipitous decline in WBC, which can occur rarely. If any of these symptoms occur, a CBC (complete blood count) should be obtained immediately.

Most patients who do well on clozapine would end up needing to be on the medication long-term for maintaining clinical improvement, because clozapine does not cure psychosis, but only controls it, similar to the use of insulin in diabetes. Another important clinical observation is that some patients become more floridly psychotic when taken off of clozapine, even after they are switched to another antipsychotic, including risperidone. When risperidone was introduced in early 1994, it was felt that risperidone would give antipsychotic efficacy similar to clozapine, without the risk of agranulocytosis and seizure and without the need for weekly CBCs. Thus, it was reasonable to consider switching patients from clozapine to risperidone. The author, following this line of reasoning, attempted to switch several patients from clozapine to risperidone with disastrous results. It is as if patients go through a period of rebound psychosis in which their psychotic symptoms such as delusions, hallucinations, and agitation, are much worse than prior to starting clozapine. Hence, any time clozapine is discontinued in a patient, gradual tapering along with close clinical supervision and monitoring are recommended. Refer to Table 15.4 for clozapine discontinuation schedule. Clozapine tends to improve tardive dyskinesia and tardive dystonia caused by traditional neuroleptics in some patients.

Clozapine is typically used for maintenance treatment on a long-term basis. Patients with chronic schizophrenia need to stay on maintenance medication indefinitely, since the risk of relapse and subsequent disruption and deterioration of functioning is great if medication is discontinued. Hence, from a clinical standpoint, the physician has to recommend that patients stay on the medication indefinitely, perhaps for life, depending on the individual case. It is perhaps a legal necessity that the drug manufacturer publications recommend that efforts should be made periodically to decrease the dose of clozapine and to discontinue the medication if possible. Conversely, clinical reasoning would indicate that the physician and the patient are taking considerable risks if clozapine is discontinued when the patient is doing well on it. In many cases, psychosis does not recur immediately after stopping the medication. A symptom-free period of weeks to months is the norm, but in the majority of cases, symptoms are bound to return within one year of stopping the medication. Clinical experience suggests that the more frequent the episodes of psychotic exacerbation, the more difficult it is to treat subsequent episodes, and the worse the prognosis. Any psychosocial gains the patient had achieved by maintaining on medication are probably wiped out by each acute exacerbation, not to mention the loss of confidence, increase in frustration, expense, and disruption of daily functioning associated with each episode of relapse. However, the patient's and family's requests to stop the medication are understandable and should be acknowledged. The physician has the responsibility to explain the advantages and disadvantages in simple terms and to strongly recommend that maintenance medication be continued. The disruption caused by a relapse can potentially lead to loss of job, prolonged disability, divorce, financial problems, loss of self-esteem, psychosocial deterioration, and more.

Given the morbidity associated with psychosis and given the superiority of clozapine in the control of psychotic symptoms, consideration should be given to clozapine as a first-line medication for patients who are likely to have a poor prognosis suggested by the following features:

- Early onset of symptoms (adolescent vs. adult)
- family history of schizophrenia
- Preexisting personality disorder among Cluster A (schizoid, schizotypal, and paranoid)
- Absence of precipitating stressors
- Preponderance of negative or deficit symptoms
- Insidious onset
- Prodromal symptoms

– Violent acting out tendencies
– Apathy or blunted affect
– Features of disorganized type or undifferentiated type
– Poor social support
– Disorganized delusions
– Chronic hostility and agitation

EFFECTIVE COMBINATIONS INVOLVING CLOZAPINE

Clozapine plus a low dose of risperidone or other high-potency non-phenothiazine antipsychotics are at times clinically necessary and effective. The possible clinical contexts in which such a combination can be successfully used include the following:

1. When initiating clozapine therapy it is frequently necessary to treat the patient using a high-potency antipsychotic during the first four to seven days or until a reasonable clozapine dose is reached, usually above 150 to 200 mg per day. Among the high-potency antipsychotics risperidone, haloperidol, and thiothixene are preferred. Phenothiazines should be avoided because of their rare effects on bone marrow.
2. If a patient derives partial and unique benefits from clozapine at a particular dose, but further needed dosage increase leads to intolerable side effects, the dose of clozapine may be kept at a tolerable dose and a high-potency antipsychotic may be added to obtain optimal benefit.
3. If seizure is a particular concern and if the patient is unable to tolerate anticonvulsants, the dose of clozapine may be reduced to a statistically safe range at which seizure risk is low (less than 400 mg per day), and a high-potency antipsychotic may be added for best results.

A benzodiazepine may be added to clozapine for treatment of insomnia or anxiety. Low doses of trazodone or nefazodone also can be added for treatment of insomnia. If depression is identified, an antidepressant, preferably one of the SSRIs, may be added. Clomipramine, bupropion, TCAs, and MAOIs are best avoided with clozapine to minimize various side effect synergism. Valproate, lamotrigine, and gabapentin are preferred for seizure prophylaxis. Clozapine can be used with lithium and valproate for treatment of manic symptoms not controlled on clozapine.

The author's general approach is first to introduce clozapine and to get the dose to a fair therapeutic range of 200 to 500 mg daily. If there are still residual symptoms that need treatment, various adjunctive medications as have been described, are then added sequentially depending on the specific needs of an individual patient. It has been a frequent clinical observation that many patients whose symptoms have barely been controlled on a combination of multiple psychotropic medications, when switched to clozapine, are able to function well on clozapine alone. Hence, the chances are that clozapine's superior and broad therapeutic effects will supersede the need for various adjunctive medications. However, treatment using clozapine alone is not sufficient for some patients; hence, combinations involving clozapine and other medications are necessary for optimal outcome. Useful combinations are listed in Table 15.3.

Weekly CBC monitoring is designed to identify the 1 percent of patients at risk for agranulocytosis. By strictly following a weekly CBC during the first year, more than 98 percent of the occurrences of bone marrow suppression can be diagnosed promptly and immediate treatment initiated, thereby considerably decreasing the chances of mortality. Furthermore, patients are routinely advised to report any signs of infection and to get an immediate CBC at the first sign or suspicion of infection. When both precautions are adhered to, the author's opinion is that mortality due to agranulocytosis can be decreased significantly.

Data on file at Sandoz Pharmaceutical Corporation revealed that there were 13 deaths due to agranulocytosis in a five-year period from February 1990 through June 1995, when 109,550 patients had taken clozapine, suggesting a mortality rate* of one death due to agranulocytosis per 8,426 patients treated with clozapine. Given the substantial risk of suicide (estimated at approximately 10 percent) among the poorly treated severely mentally ill patients, the mortality rate if not treated with clozapine is expected to be much higher

*In this context, mortality rate is intended to mean a general index of risk or probability of death.

TABLE 15.3. Medications That Can Be Combined with Clozapine

Residual Symptoms	Medications to Add to Clozapine
Depression	antidepressants; SSRIs preferred
Anxiety	benzodiazepines preferred*
"Positive" symptoms of psychosis	high-potency antipsychotics; risperidone preferred (low dose of depot haloperidol decanoate may improve noncompliance and residual "positive" symptoms)
Extreme mood instability	lithium, valproic acid, lamotrigine, gabapentin
Marked anergia	stimulants, caffeine
Obsessive-compulsive symptoms	antiobsessional medications; SSRIs preferred
Substance abuse	naltrexone

*Watch for respiratory depression or excessive sedation when a benzodiazepine and clozapine are given concurrently during the first week of initiation of clozapine in the elderly. After the first week, coadministration of a benzodiazepine has been well tolerated by the elderly, in the author's experience.

than the mortality rate due to agranulocytosis, making clozapine treatment of the severely ill safer than not treating with clozapine. Assuming a 10 percent mortality rate due to suicide among the poorly treated chronically psychotic patient population, it can be estimated that there would be 10,950 suicides (10 percent of 109,550 patients) if all 109,550 patients had treatment-refractory illness and if clozapine was not made available to these patients. This can be compared to 13 deaths attributed directly to clozapine among 109,550 patients on clozapine therapy. Although there are other confounding variables including availability of risperidone and prolonged inpatient hospitalization as options that can alter the analysis described above, it is clear that clozapine still has a favorable benefit-to-risk ratio despite the risk of fatality as a result of agranulocytosis.

Given the probability that most patients with schizophrenia and schizoaffective disorder eventually develop treatment-resistance when treated long enough on traditional antipsychotic agents, "treatment-resistance" may be considered one of the characteristics of schizophrenia or one of the inherent long-term consequences of treatment using traditional antipsychotic agents, supporting the clinical wisdom of considering the use of clozapine as a first-line treatment option for selected patients expected to need long-term antipsychotic therapy.

Traditional antipsychotics cause numerous side effects such as extrapyramidal symptoms and increased risk of tardive dyskinesia. In addition, they do not satisfactorily treat negative symptoms; hence, compliance is a perennial problem. Although risperidone is superior to traditional antipsychotics in this regard and therefore should be preferred over traditional antipsychotics, the author's experience indicates that clozapine is superior to even risperidone and much superior to traditional antipsychotics. If a patient presents with several of the poor prognosticators, there are many clinical reasons, as outlined above, notwithstanding cost considerations, to consider clozapine as the first-line antipsychotic for long-term maintenance if the diagnosis is schizophrenia or schizoaffective disorder.

A cost analysis indicates that to maintain a patient on haloperidol 5 mg daily (which is a reasonable maintenance dose), the monthly cost is expected to average $8; even when an adjunctive anticholinergic such as benzotropine mesylate 1 mg BID is needed, the total cost for a month's supply of medications is likely to be approximately $18. This can be compared to the cost of $175 per month for risperidone 2 mg BID and $220 per month for olanzapine 10 mg HS, which are reasonable maintenance doses. The cost of maintaining on clozapine 300 mg daily (which should be a reasonable maintenance dose in clinical practice), including the cost of weekly CBCs at $15 per CBC, should be approximately $370 per month. Although the cost savings with the use of haloperidol are considerable compared to olanzapine, risperidone, and clozapine, any significant overall clinical advantage to the patient suffering from such a debilitating illness should be worth the additional cost, both from a humane perspective and from a long-term economic impact perspective. An illness or symptom that is not so debilitating probably deserves more attention to cost considerations. For example, temazepam (Restoril) 15 mg costs $7 per month, whereas zolpidem (Ambien) 10 mg costs $50 per month. Both of these medications can be used for short-term treatment of insomnia. In this example, even though zolpidem is superior to temazepam for initial insomnia, the cost difference in excess of $40 per month is significant, given the clinical observation that both treat insomnia fairly well. Hence, the clinically and economically prudent strategy is to prescribe the least expensive medication for the treatment of fairly inconsequential symptoms. It follows, then, that it is equally prudent to prescribe the most superior medication obtainable for one of the most debilitating of medical conditions, schizophrenia, despite the high cost.

DISCONTINUATION OF CLOZAPINE

It is generally not prudent to discontinue clozapine if it is effective. However, clozapine may have to be discontinued in the following contexts.

1. Clozapine is not effective.
2. Clozapine side effects prevent continued treatment.
3. Maintenance on clozapine is difficult due to economic or other reasons.
4. The patient decides to discontinue clozapine for whatever reason.

In ideal conditions clozapine should be gradually tapered off at a rate of 10 to 15 percent decrease daily, over a span of 10 to 20 days, while the patient is being introduced to the new antipsychotic. Prior to the conclusion of the clozapine taper, the new antipsychotic should be at the optimal therapeutic dose to prevent relapse of psychosis. Rapid discontinuation of clozapine can lead to a "rebound psychosis," characterized by confusion, agitation, mania, paranoia, hyperactivity, insomnia, auditory and visual hallucinations, loose associations, and even disorientation, necessitating immediate hospitalization. The rebound psychosis may require treatment using sedating medications, including low-potency antipsychotics and benzodiazepines. Clinical experience indicates that patients who had a superior response to clozapine and who were on doses higher than 300 mg daily tend to develop rebound psychosis more frequently compared to those who did not respond well to clozapine. Obviously, some clozapine side effects require immediate discontinuation due to medical reasons, e.g., agranulocytosis, cardiorespiratory abnormalities, and severe hypotension, in which case the patient should be closely monitored for the development of rebound psychosis. Occasionally, hospitalization may be considered for safe and rapid withdrawal from clozapine. Rebound psychosis is managed in the same manner as acute psychosis.

A sample schedule for the elective discontinuation of clozapine of a patient maintained on clozapine 400 mg daily is given in Table 15.4. If clozapine is discontinued due to lack of efficacy, the patient may tolerate a more rapid discontinuation rate. The drug manufacturer recommends weekly WBC monitoring for four weeks after clozapine has been stopped.

TABLE 15.4 Clozapine: Elective Discontinuation Schedule

Day	Total Dose/Day
0	400 mg (maintenance dose)
1	350 mg
2	300 mg
3	250 mg
4	200 mg
5	175 mg
6	150 mg
7	125 mg
8	100 mg
9	75 mg
10	50 mg
11	25 mg
12	25 mg
13	12.5 mg
14	12.5 mg

TECHNIQUES TO DETECT OR MINIMIZE SERIOUS CLOZAPINE SIDE EFFECTS

Agranulocytosis

Since most occurrences of agranulocytosis are reported between two weeks and four months of initiation of clozapine, clinicians or patients who want to be extra cautious may choose to obtain a WBC more frequently than required by the drug manufacturer. For example, the WBC could be obtained every Monday and Friday during the most vulnerable period. After the first four months, the frequency of WBC monitoring may be decreased to the minimum required weekly schedule.

Seizures

Since seizure risk is dose-dependent, it is prudent to consider a prophylactic anticonvulsant for patients who need to be on more than 500 mg of clozapine per day. The seizure risk at this dose or higher is estimated at 5 percent. It is likely that the seizure risk is greater than 5 percent at a dose of 900 mg per day, which is the maximum approved dose of clozapine. Valproate, lamotrigine (Lamictal), or gabapentin (Neurontin) are preferred for seizure prophylaxis. An EEG (after the clozapine dosage has been stabilized) can be obtained to rule out the presence of subclinical seizure activity, and may be desirable if clozapine dose exceeds 500 mg per day. Carbamazepine and phenytoin are best avoided due to possible additive effects on bone marrow.

Respiratory Depression and Respiratory Collapse

Avoid benzodiazepines early in treatment, especially when clozapine is first administered. Give a low dose of clozapine (12.5 mg) on the first day, particularly for the elderly. Institute slow dosage escalation if sedation is a problem. A benzodiazepine may be safely introduced after the clozapine dosage escalation is completed.

Management of various side effects such as hypersalivation, excessive sedation, dizziness, fever, leukocytosis, etc., is described in a booklet published by Sandoz, *Clozaril–Management of Adverse Events,* and is presented in summarized and modified form in Table 15.7. Table 15.5 lists common adverse events related to clozapine. WBC-related adverse events and suggested actions are summarized in Table 15.6. Table 15.7 lists common side effects and specific management suggestions in a chart format.

TABLE 15.5. Adverse Effects Related to Clozapine

Serious Events	Other Events
agranulocytosis hypotension, cardiac arrest, respiratory depression	sedation dizziness seizure salvation tachycardia weight gain fever constipation hypotension nausea/vomiting headache leukocytosis

Source: *Clozaril–Management of Adverse Effects.* 1993. Sandoz Pharmaceuticals.

STARTING CLOZAPINE–TO HOSPITALIZE OR NOT

In principle, clozapine can be started on an outpatient basis. Patients who are not acutely symptomatic, are in control, and are reliable are particularly good candidates for consideration for initiation of clozapine on an outpatient basis. However, the practical reality is that in most cases, those patients who are selected for clozapine therapy are acutely symptomatic with florid symptoms that are poorly controlled on traditional antipsychotic medications. These patients typically need inpatient treatment regardless of clozapine initiation. Patients

TABLE 15.6. White Blood Cell Count/Granulocyte-Related Events and Suggested Actions

	WBC Count/Granulocyte	Actions
Screening	Before treatment: WBC<3,500/mcl	Treatment not initiated Other contraindications: Myeloproliferative disorders Previous Clozaril-induced agranulocytosis or severe granulocytopenia Simultaneous use with other agents having a well-known potential to suppress bone marrow function.
	WBC>3,500/mcl No previous agranulocytosis	Initiate treatment.
Normal WBC results	After Clozaril treatment initiated: WBC>3,500/mcl, no substantial drop from baseline	Continue treatment with weekly WBC testing and drug dispensing.
Mild Leukopenia	WBC<3,500/mcl or substantial drop in baseline, even if WBC>3,500/mcl or immature forms present	1. Repeat WBC and do differential count; continue twice-weekly WBC and differential until WBC exceeds 3,500/mcl.
Moderate Leukopenia	After action 1: Total WBC<3,000/mcl or granulocyte count is <1,500/mcl	2. Interrupt therapy; institute daily WBC and differential counts, monitor patient for flu-like symptoms or other symptoms of infection.

	WBC Count/Granulocyte	Actions
Moderate Leukopenia (Continued)	If after action 2: No symptoms of infection develop	3A. Resume Clozaril therapy.*
	Total WBC returns to levels >3,000/mcl Granulocytes return to levels >1,500/mcl	Continue twice-weekly WBC and differential counts until total WBC counts return to levels >3,500/mcl.
Severe Leukopenia or Agranulocytosis	WBC falls to <2,000/mcl or granulocytes fall to <1,000/mcl	3B. Consider bone marrow aspiration to ascertain granulopoietic status.
	Granulocytes fall to <500/mcl	If granulopoiesis is deficient, protective isolation may be indicated. Consider treatment using Granulocyte Colony Stimulating Factor such as filgrastin (Neupogen). If evidence of infection develops, take appropriate cultures and start patient on appropriate antibiotic regimen. Do not rechallenge with Clozaril. Continue WBC counts for four consecutive weeks after discontinuation of Clozaril.

Notes: Granulocyte defined as bands plus polys (absolute neutrophil count)

*When patients who have been off Clozaril for two days or longer are restarted, it is recommended that treatment be initiated with one-half of a 25 mg tablet (12.5 mg)

Source: Table modified from Sandoz Pharmaceuticals: *Clozaril–Management of Adverse Events,* 1993. Used with permission.

TABLE 15.7. Clozapine Side Effect Management Chart

Side Effects	Management Suggestions
Seizures: Grand Mal, myoclonic jerks, and cataleptic-like events. Preexisting seizure disorder is not a contraindication to clozapine. Can occur at any time. 5 percent risk for doses > 500 mg per day. Increased risk in patients with history of closed head injury.	Avoid rapid dosage escalation. Use divided doses (TID). Avoid combining with other drugs that lower seizure threshold. Do EEG, neurological consultation. Decrease dose. Start anticonvulsant for treatment of seizures. Avoid carbamazepine/ phenytoin. Consider prophylactic anticonvulsant if dosage exceeds 500 mg per day.
Hypotension: Systolic blood pressure < 90 mm Hg. Occurs in 9 percent; more common in elderly. Collapse occurs in 1 in 3,000. Can occur in the first four weeks. May subside over time.	Avoid rapid dosage escalation. Monitor blood pressure and pulse QID supine and standing. Instruct patient to stand slowly. Start first dose at 12.5 mg. Give major dose at bedtime; wear support stockings. Avoid concurrent benzodiazepines. If persistent and severe, consider fludrocortisone acetate 0.1 mg BID-TID with medical clearance and monitoring. Avoid epinephrine because of possible reverse epinephrine effects.
Sedation/Drowsiness: Presents with weakness, fatigue, lethargy, and hypersomnia. Occurs in 30 to 35 percent in the first four weeks. May improve over time.	Give major portion at bedtime. Increase dose slowly. Avoid activities requiring alertness. Add caffeine. Avoid other sedating drugs. For severe sedation, may try dextroamphetamine 5 to 10 mg or methylphenidate 5 to 10 mg AM and noon.
Dizziness/Vertigo: A sensation of unsteadiness with a feeling of movement within the head or external world. Occurs in 19 percent. Can occur at any time during treatment, usually as a result of orthostatic hypotension. Elderly patients are at particular risk while therapy is being initiated.	Slow dosage titration. Monitor blood pressure supine and standing. Advise patient to stand up slowly from sitting or lying positions. Caution while engaging in activities requiring balance and coordination.
Hypersalivation: Can be profuse during sleep. Occurs in 40 percent. Appears within four weeks. May subside over time.	Prop up pillow. Encourage patients to sleep on their side, use a towel to cover pillow. If severe, consider an anticholinergic or clonidine transdermal patch 0.1 to 0.2 mg/week temporarily.

Side Effects	Management Suggestions
Tachycardia: Heart rate > 120 per minute, or heart rate > 100 per minute and patient is symptomatic (sweating, dizziness, chest pain), or coronary risk factors present. Early in treatment, can persist. Tolerance can develop.	Avoid rapid dosage escalation. Reduce caffeine intake and cigarette smoking. If asymptomatic, with no coronary risk factors (obesity, hypertension, smoking, diabetes, family history of CAD, or previous history of CAD), observe two weeks. If patient is younger than 30 years old, is healthy, with no medical problems or CAD risk factors, and no contra-indications to beta-blockers (asthma, bronchospastic disease, diabetes, hypoglycemia), can begin atenolol (Tenormin) 25 to 50 mg per day. If tachycardia persists, switch to pindolol (Visken) 5 mg po QD. May increase to 5 mg BID, then 10 mg BID, if necessary. Cardiac evaluation to rule out heart disease. Reduce clozapine dose if other interventions not effective.
Constipation: Occurs in 15 percent. Dose-dependent. May improve over time. Rarely, can progress to obstipation or ileus.	High fiber diet. Eliminate other anticholinergic drugs. Increase fluid intake, encourage physical activity. Docusate sodium (Colase) 200 to 300 mg per day. Psyllium hydrophilic mucilloid (Metamucil) one dose per day. Vigorous early treatment can prevent complications.
Fever: May last three to five days. Occurs in the first three weeks. Usually benign. Temperature >100.4 degrees F (38 degrees C). Occurs in 10 percent.	Rule out infection; rule out agranulocytosis. For temperature >102 degrees F, rule out NMS. Medical consultation if fever is severe or persistent. Symptomatic treatment using aspirin or acetaminophen. Continue clozapine dosage; increase if fever is benign.
Weight Gain: Can be from 2 to 25 pounds and persistent. Occurs in about 15 percent. More common in younger patients.	Exercise, watch diet, dietary counseling. If severe and persistent, consider cautious trial on low doses of fenfluramine at 10 to 20 mg two hours AC supper.

TABLE 15.7 (continued)

Side Effects	Management Suggestions
Leukocytosis: low incidence. Appears within first four to eight weeks and gradually subsides. Can be dose-dependent.	Rule out infection, medical illness, eosinophilia, NMS, and other etiologies of leukocytosis. Usually benign. Dosage decrease may improve leukocytosis. Continue to monitor for infection.
Headache: Occurs in 7 percent. Transient, subsides over time.	Analgesic treatment. If persistent, rule out other causes.
Hypertension: Frequency 4 percent. Blood pressure >150/90 mm Hg. Usually dose-dependent.	Avoid rapid dosage escalation. Monitor blood pressure four times a day for two weeks. If significant, initiate antihypertensive therapy (atenolol 50 to 100 mg per day, or pindolol 5 to 10 mg BID). Avoid ACE inhibitors, which have been associated with agranulocytosis.
Nausea/Vomiting: Occurs after four to six weeks.	Reduce the dose and titrate more slowly. If severe, give trimethobenzamide (Tigan), or metoclopramide (Reglan), or prochlorperazine (Compazine). Supplement fluids via IV route if unable to take fluids orally. Check BUN, creatinine, and electrolytes if vomiting is severe and persists more than 48 hours.
Urinary Problems: Frequency 6 percent. Incontinence, enuresis, increased frequency and urgency, hesitancy, and urinary retention. Usually improves over time. Can be dose-dependent.	For incontinence, consider anticholinergic drugs for urologic applications; for urinary hesitancy and retention, consider bethanechol. Consider desmopressin nasal spray for enuresis.
Delirium/Confusion: Disorientation, confusion, worse at night. Can be dose-dependent.	Rule out medical etiology and polypharmacy. Consider EEG. Rule out anticholinergic toxicity. Decrease clozapine dose.

Source: Adapted with modifications from Sandoz Corporation: "Clozaril Side Effect Management Chart," *Clozaril Treatment Trends* 4(1) 1995. Used with permission. Table includes data and recommendations derived from the author's clinical experience.

whose symptoms are stabilized on a traditional antipsychotic and who have intolerable side effects attributed to traditional antipsychotics are another group of patients who could benefit from clozapine treatment. The process of tapering off the traditional antipsychotic and of initiating clozapine involves many medical aspects, some of which are listed below:

- There is a likelihood of relapse if the existing antipsychotic is abruptly stopped or rapidly tapered off.
- A relapse might make the patient immediately noncompliant, resulting in further deterioration.
- A careful titration of clozapine dose, with frequent monitoring of vital signs, is essential during the first three to six days to enhance the chances of successful outcome.
- The clozapine dose cannot be rapidly increased should the patient become acutely psychotic, necessitating immediate intervention that is difficult for the outpatient.
- Though ideally clozapine is to be used as a single medication, in actual clinical practice most patients need adjunctive medications (including adjunctive low-dose high-potency traditional antipsychotics or a low dose of risperidone) for optimal outcome. This is crucial during the first several days of clozapine initiation.
- The most common side effects of clozapine such as dizziness, tachycardia, nausea, hypersalivation, sedation, constipation, and orthostatic changes need medical supervision, management, and frequent reassurance to overcome or to be tolerated by the patient.
- The clozapine titration schedule during the first three to six days is fairly complex. An example of a fairly rapid initiation schedule is given below:

	AM	Noon	PM	HS
Day 1	–	12.5 mg	12.5 mg	12.5 mg
Day 2	12.5	12.5	25	25
Day 3	25	25	25	50
Day 4	25	25	50	75
Day 5	25	25	50	100

Obviously, any major side effects or complications necessitate a slower schedule. A slower schedule still is fairly complex with an increased risk of relapse. As is evident, such a schedule would be very difficult for a seriously ill psychiatric patient to comply with as an outpatient, during the initiation phase.

- The dose of the existing traditional antipsychotic preferably should not be abruptly discontinued, but must be gradually tapered off. An example:

	Haloperidol Dose
Day 1	10 mg HS
Day 2	8 mg HS
Day 3	6 mg HS
Day 4	4 mg HS
Day 5	2 mg HS, then discontinue

  Again, severely and chronically mentally ill patients who are fairly dysfunctional (patients who comprise the clozapine target group) will have great difficulty in adhering to these complex schedules during the clozapine initiation phase.
- If the existing antipsychotic is of low potency (such as chlorpromazine or thioridazine), it should preferably be discontinued before clozapine can be introduced for medical reasons (such as risk of hypotension, excessive sedation, and cardiorespiratory problems), thereby increasing the chances of the patient becoming symptomatic during the first three to six days that are necessary to get the clozapine dose to a low therapeutic range of 100 to 200 mg.
- Highly skilled clinical measures such as reassurance, support, persuasion, insistence, perseverance, and close attention to detail are typically needed during the first three to six days to get many patients to complete the clozapine titration process. Some patients may even require emergency intervention to control agitation, including seclusion and restraints during clozapine initiation phase.
- The complex clozapine titration schedule and the gradual tapering off schedule of the existing antipsychotic are difficult for most severely mentally ill patients to implement as outpatients unless supportive, responsible, and capable family members or

clinical staff are available to closely supervise the treatment in an outpatient setting.

- Many complications and problems, some of which are listed above, can threaten the chance of a successful outpatient clozapine initiation process, leading to the erroneous conclusion that clozapine was either ineffective or intolerable, when proper clozapine treatment as an inpatient could overcome most of the initial complications, thereby enhancing the chance of a successful outcome.
- Poor initiation could lead to improper abandonment of clozapine, which could have been a potentially life-saving therapeutic intervention.
- Clozapine initiation as an outpatient would have to be fairly slow to avoid medical risks. However, slow initiation places the patient at high risk for a relapse, which will require control of the acute relapse and all of the complications associated with a relapse, such as refusal to accept treatment, need for involuntary proceedings, refusal of clozapine, and a greater risk of suicide, among others. Obviously, a longer period of hospitalization would generally be required should the patient experience a relapse.

Initiating clozapine can be compared to initiating insulin therapy for a newly diagnosed Type I diabetic. Diabetes will have varying degrees of "brittleness," and this creates different levels of difficulty in controlling each patient's basic disease process. Diabetic patients have varying insulin requirements; therefore, adjusting their dosage based on frequent blood sugar monitoring becomes a quite active and critical clinical process. If done poorly, dosage adjustment can result in harmful extremes of hypoglycemia and/or ketoacidosis. Prescription of a compatible diet is also important. Proper management of complications and absence of negative experiences during the introduction of insulin therapy enhance compliance. A successful initiation of insulin greatly improves the chances of avoiding future complications and hospitalizations. For these clinical reasons, insulin therapy is typically initiated as an inpatient. Once insulin is properly initiated, subsequent management can be safely carried out as an outpatient. As a final comparison, a poor initiation of insulin therapy does not result in abandonment of that therapy, whereas regarding clozapine, a poor initiation is likely to result in a false conclusion that clozapine was not effective, and the patient will forever abandon a possibly life-saving therapy.

In the author's experience, clozapine is a superior medication for the treatment of selected severely mentally ill psychiatric patients. To take full advantage of its unique benefits without letting the many side effects defeat the treatment, it has to be introduced to the patient appropriately. When clozapine is initiated in an inpatient setting, in the author's estimate, the chance of a successful outcome is in the 70 to 80 percent range; if it is started in an outpatient setting, the chance of successful outcome is lower. In most cases, three to eight days of inpatient stay is sufficient to get the patient to a dose of 100 to 200 mg, with further dosage titration safely and easily conducted on an outpatient basis. The author has virtually stopped the practice of starting clozapine in an outpatient setting due to the unsatisfactory results.

To begin a patient on clozapine as an outpatient in the interest of economy would be penny-wise and pound-foolish, in most cases. In strict financial terms clozapine treatment is expensive in the short-term, but cost effective in the long-term. When there is such a flux in the health insurance industry as is evident currently with frequent changes of insurance carriers, utilization review incentives for maximum cost savings and competitive bidding for utilization review contracts where the focus is on immediate profit, it would make no business sense for profit-oriented third-party payers to enthusiastically endorse clozapine therapy. The treating clinician has become the only professional to advocate for the patients' best interests, both short- and long-term.

In summary, for assuring the best outcome, it is recommended that, for the majority of patients, clozapine be initiated in an inpatient setting as a general medical practice, regardless of whether or not patients are willing to start clozapine as outpatients.

Summary of Advantages and Disadvantages of Clozapine

Advantages

- Superior effectiveness for positive symptoms of psychoses
- The most effective among currently available antipsychotics for negative symptoms

– Virtual absence of tardive dyskinesia
– May cause regression of tardive dyskinesia and tardive dystonia induced by traditional antipsychotics
– Extremely low incidence of extrapyramidal symptoms and neuroleptic malignant syndrome
– Has antianxiety, antidepressant, and mood-stabilizer properties
– Effective for controlling psychotic symptoms regardless of diagnosis; may be used in schizophrenia, schizoaffective disorder, severe bipolar disorder, delusional disorder, major depression with psychotic features, or any disorder with chronic psychotic symptoms as listed in the text
– Superior results can eventually enhance insight and compliance, and improve overall patient functioning and quality of life
– Improvement tends to continue for up to six months, or longer, prior to reaching a plateau
– Does not elevate prolactin level; low incidence of galactorrhea, gynecomastia, and amenorrhea; since it is estimated that about one-third of human breast cancer is prolactin sensitive, there may be at least a theoretical advantage in using clozapine in patients with a history of breast cancer or in those who are predisposed to it
– Sedating properties may help insomnia, a common problem in psychotic patients
– Clozapine can supplant the need for a variety of adjunctive medications such as mood stabilizers, anticholinergics, antidepressants, and benzodiazepines, suggesting that clozapine has a broad spectrum of therapeutic effects
– Satisfactory response to clozapine substantially reduces risk of suicide attempts
– Clozapine could reduce the craving for and abuse of drugs, alcohol, and nicotine frequently found among psychotic patients
– Striking decrease in relapse and rehospitalization rate
– FDA pregnancy category B

Disadvantages

– 1 percent incidence of agranulocytosis and consequent need for weekly CBC monitoring for detection of neutropenia; slightly greater risk in females and in geriatric patients; greatest risk is in the first four months of initiating clozapine treatment

- 4 to 5 percent risk of seizures at higher doses, compared to 1 percent risk of seizures with other antipsychotics
- High cost of treatment (average of $5,500 per year on a dose of 350 mg per day and for weekly CBCs)
- Initiation of treatment may require inpatient stay in most cases for optimal outcome (which can be accomplished in three to eight days)
- Parenteral or liquid form not available in the United States
- In some patients, sedation and orthostatic hypotension can be excessive, preventing increase to therapeutic range
- Relatively greater incidence of tachycardia, hypotension, and hypersalivation
- One death (due to agranulocytosis) per 8,426 patients treated with clozapine
- Side effects such as somnolence, weight gain, anergia, and a "drugged" feeling can be persistent in some patients

Administrative Disadvantages

High initial and maintenance cost can be a disincentive to many community mental health centers (CMHC) that have limited budgets but care for a high percentage of patients with chronic mental illness, which is a subgroup of patients who significantly benefit from clozapine. Administrators realize that funding decisions are made and their own accomplishments judged based on short-term and immediate budgetary performance, as is true with regard to most business practices. Any cost savings due to a decreased number of readmissions expected from clozapine treatment is likely to be realized only years later. Improvement in the patient's quality of life is difficult to quantify. Often unrecognized, it is likely to occur gradually and slowly after initiation of clozapine treatment. Since there is a considerable turnover of administrators of CMHCs, the person who makes the decision today to allocate funding for clozapine treatment is not likely to receive any recognition for long-term cost savings. In fact, if clozapine treatment causes short-term budgetary constraints, which is quite possible during the first several years, it may adversely reflect on the administrator. Moreover, in most cases any cost savings in the long run will not be realized by the CMHC, but will benefit the state and federal agencies that administer inpatient health insurance for the indigent. To use an analogy, clozapine is like a long-term investment, and hence is unlikely to appeal to short-term investors who are looking for quick returns. All of these factors make it difficult for administrators of CMHCs to become enthusiastic about clozapine, unless policy makers have the foresight and wisdom to allocate to CMHCs at least a portion of the cost savings expected to result from reduced hospitalization rate, for funding the higher initiation, maintenance and patient monitoring costs associated with clozapine therapy.

Another factor is that some inpatient units that are dependent on readmissions of chronic patients, are likely to suffer in the long term with clozapine treatment, due to decreased patient census resulting from clozapine's established efficacy in reducing rehospitalization rate. Therefore, strictly from an administrator's standpoint, those inpatient units which primarily rely on treating chronic patients could have potential long term losses by encouraging clozapine. Those who need a reason to discourage clozapine use have agranulocytosis risk to cite as an apparently rational argument against clozapine.

In summary, clozapine is a superior medication for the treatment of a variety of chronic psychotic conditions and selected chronic severe mental disorders. It is a complicated medication that requires skillful initiation and careful clinical management. Weekly WBC monitoring enables early detection and treatment of agranulocytosis, preventing a fatal outcome in the great majority of patients. Seizure prophylaxis significantly decreases the seizure risk associated with clozapine dose in the higher dosage range. Clozapine treatment significantly decreases suicide risk. The benefits of clozapine therapy far outweigh the risks associated with it.

OLANZAPINE (ZYPREXA)

Olanzapine, an atypical antipsychotic with serotonin-dopamine antagonist (SDA) effects, was introduced in the United States in October 1996. It is available as unscored 5 mg, 7.5 mg, and 10 mg tablets. The elimination half-life is 30 hours. Plasma-protein binding is 95 percent. The major metabolic route is hepatic, necessitating dosage adjustment in the hepatically impaired and in the elderly. The starting dose as well as the optimal dose recommended by the drug manufacturer for treatment of schizophrenia is 10 mg daily. The dosage range is from 5 to 20 mg daily. All or a major portion of the dose may be given at bedtime to enhance sleep and to minimize daytime drowsiness.

Olanzapine is well tolerated by most patients. Many patients reported significant anxiolytic and calming effects. Its low risk of EPS, effectiveness for both positive and negative symptoms, and absence of major side effects should make it a superior antipsychotic compared to traditional antipsychotics. Furthermore, it does not elevate serum prolactin level significantly, an advantage also shared by clozapine and sertindole, but not by risperidone, among the atypical antipsychotics. Since clinical experience so far has sustantiated the expectation particularly of fair effectiveness in treating negative symptoms, low EPS, a benign side effect profile, minimal effects on prolactin level, and superior tolerability, olanzapine has the potential to be the first-line general purpose antipsychotic of choice for treatment of schizophrenia and psychotic symptoms.

The common side effects reported for olanzapine are drowsiness, lightheadedness, dry mouth, weight gain, anxiety, edema, and orthostatic hypotension. Most of these side effects typically subside within one to two weeks of starting the medication. However, some weight gain is likely to persist for the duration of olanzapine therapy. Olanzapine can trigger mania. Rare incidence of hepatotoxicity has also been reported. Therefore, monitoring of liver function after two weeks and a repeat test after two months of starting olanzapine may be performed in patients susceptible to live enzyme elevation such as patients with hepatic disease or patients who are being treated with potentially hepatotoxic drugs. Most cases of liver enzyme elevations are transient and tend to subside without the need for dosage adjustment. Liver function studies or laboratory tests are neither necessary nor recommended on a routine basis.

Since orthostatic hypotension associated with dizziness and syncope can occur in rare patients, the author's practice is to start patients on olanzapine 5 mg and increase to 10 mg after two to three days, particularly for outpatients. A lower starting dose of 2.5 mg or 3.75 mg may be considered for patients with cardiovascular disease and cerebrovascular disease, and for patients taking antihypertensive medications.

Since clinical experience suggests possible effectiveness for treatment of some treatment-resistant schizophrenias, olanzapine could be a treatment option prior to a trial of clozapine, which, for general purpose use, is fettered by a 1 to 2 percent risk of argranulocytosis.

As is generally the case with most psychiatric conditions, mild symptoms might respond to low doses and severe and chronic symptoms might need doses at the higher end of the therapeutic range. Olanzapine dosage guidelines based on the author's clinical experience are given below.

Olanzapine Dosage Guidelines

- Conditions with mild psychotic symptoms such as paranoid personality features, schizotypal features, schizoid features, and dementia might respond to doses in the range of 1.25 to 5 mg daily
- Conditions with moderate psychotic symptoms such as delusional disorders, psychotic symptoms associated with affective disorders, schizoaffective disorders, and bipolar disorder might respond to a dosage range of 5 to 10 mg daily
- Conditions characterized by severe psychotic symptoms such as the schizophrenias and severe schizoaffective disorder might need a dosage range of 10 to 20 mg daily for adequate response

Adjunctive Medications

SSRIs, MAOIs, TCAs, bupropion, mirtazapine, trazodone, nefazodone, lithium, valproate, carbamazepine, gabapentin, lamotrigine, and the benzodiazepines may be employed if necessary in a combination treatment regimen involving olanzapine.

Antipsychotic Combinations Involving Olanzapine

Some patients may require the adjunctive use of other antipsychotics for optimal symptom control if olanzapine alone is not sufficient to provide satisfactory control of symptoms. It should be emphasized that as a general rule, polypharmacy should be avoided unless necessary and beneficial to the patient. Antipsychotic combinations involving clozapine and risperidone are not uncommon. Low doses of risperidone or traditional antipsychotics can be combined with a therapeutic dose of olanzapine to control breakthrough psychotic symptoms if olanzapine is otherwise well tolerated or provides other unique and significant benefits to the patient. When multiple medications are employed, the patient is at risk for developing side effects from each of the medications independently and additively. The author has no experience in combining olanzapine and clozapine, but it is conceivable that a rare patient may benefit from such a combination.

Whether or Not to Switch to Olanzapine

The general clinical strategy is not to switch if the patient is doing well on clozapine or risperidone, both of which have low risk of causing tardive dyskinesia; however, in the case of risperidone, the TD risk is considered greater than that of clozapine, but less than that of traditional antipsychotics. Patients who have responded particularly well to clozapine tend to do poorly when switched to other antipsychotics. Therefore, patients functioning well on clozapine should be switched only if necessary and not simply to try a new antipsychotic. The author's practice is to attempt to switch patients taking traditional antipsychotics to atypical antipsychotics even if they are currently doing well because of the inherent potential of traditional antipsychotics to cause TD in a significant proportion of patients after chronic use. Why wait for TD to emerge when it could be irreversible? Atypical antipsychotics including olanzapine offer the theoretical probability of low risk of TD. Since olanzapine tends to cause less acute EPS compared to traditional antipsychotics and since olanzapine does not have the leukopenic and epileptogenic potential of clozapine, olanzapine should be a strong candidate for choice as a first-line agent or an agent to switch patients to, among the currently available atypical antipsychotics, all of which have various advantages over the traditional antipsychotics as discussed in the sections describing each of the antipsychotics individually. Clozapine is expected to retain its position as the drug of choice for truly treatment-resistant schizophrenia.

Switching from Other Antipsychotics to Olanzapine

In general, gradual taper of the existing antipsychotic and concurrent gradual initiation of olanzapine is the preferred method. If the antipsychotic being discontinued has anticholinergic effects, as do for example, chlorpromazine, thioridazine, or clozapine, a slow taper over 7 to 14 days is recommended on an outpatient basis. Adjunctive anticholinergic medication is preferably discontinued over the four to six day period after starting olanzapine. If the patient has been taking a low dose of an antipsychotic in the high-potency category (for example, haloperidol 0.5 to 2 mg, thiothixene 1 to 4 mg, or equivalent), the patient may be safely switched to olanzapine without the need for gradual taper. However, low-potency antipsychotics such as chlorpromazine, thioridazine, and clozapine are preferably tapered off even if the patient has been taking a low dose (for example, chlorpromazine 25 to 75 mg or equivalent). Several switching schedules involving a few of the common antipsychotics are given below:

Haloperidol 10 mg Daily to Olanzapine

	Haloperidol	*Olanzapine*
Day 1	5 mg	5 mg
Day 2	2.5 mg	5 mg
Day 3	2.5 mg	10 mg
Day 4	1 mg	10 mg
Day 5	--	10 mg

Chlorpromazine 300 mg Daily to Olanzapine

	Chlorpromazine	*Olanzapine*
Day 1	200 mg	5 mg
Day 2	150 mg	5 mg
Day 3	100 mg	5 mg
Day 4	75 mg	10 mg
Day 5	50 mg	10 mg

Day 6	25 mg	10 mg
Day 7	--	10 mg

Clozapine 300 mg Daily to Olanzapine

	Clozapine	*Olanzapine*
Day 1	200 mg	5 mg
Day 2	150 mg	5 mg
Day 3	100 mg	5 mg
Day 4	100 mg	10 mg
Day 5	75 mg	10 mg
Day 6	75 mg	10 mg
Day 7	50 mg	10 mg
Day 8	50 mg	10 mg
Day 9	25 mg	10 mg
Day 10	25 mg	10 mg
Day 11	12.5 mg	10 mg
Day 12	12.5 mg	10 mg
Day 13	12.5 mg	10 mg
Day 14	--	10 mg

These switching schedules may be used as flexible guidelines primarily for outpatient applications. The switch may be completed more rapidly in an inpatient setting. For instance, for an inpatient the switch from haloperidol can be made by stopping haloperidol and starting olanzapine 10 mg from Day 1. Low-potency antipsychotics such as chlorpromazine and clozapine may be tapered off in four and six days, respectively, as an inpatient while olanzapine is increased to the therapeutic dose of 10 mg daily starting on Day 3. The obvious advantage for an inpatient is that if rebound psychosis, cholinergic rebound, or agitation emerge, immediate intervention can be initiated without risking noncompliance, deterioration, or other complications, whereas in the case of an outpatient, slow tapering of the existing antipsychotic and rapid titration of olanzapine to the therapeutic dose minimizes complications from drug withdrawal. Since clozapine tends to cause moderate to severe withdrawal symptoms if abruptly or rapidly discontinued, clozapine should ideally be tapered off slowly and gradually over a 10- to 20-day period depending on the total daily clozapine dose to avoid withdrawal complications. If the patient, a supportive family member, or a day program staff member is not able to supervise the slow clozapine taper and olanzapine titration as an outpatient, inpatient hospitalization should be considered, particularly if the existing clozapine dose is greater than 200 mg daily. It has to be emphasized, however, that olanzapine is not a substitute for clozapine, and that patients who have shown good response to clozapine and are tolerating clozapine well may do poorly when switched to currently available antipsychotics including olanzapine.

Cost Comparison

Olanzapine 10 mg daily, which is probably the most common dosage for treating schizophrenia, costs approximately $220 per month and $2,640 per year, compared to risperidone 2 mg BID costing approximately $180 per month and $2,160 per year, and clozapine 300 mg daily costing approximately $4,500 per year including the cost of weekly CBC. If a patient needs olanzapine 15 mg daily, which may not be uncommon, the cost would rise to approximately $325 per month and $3,900 per year. Olanzapine 10 mg daily, risperidone 2 mg BID, and clozapine 300 mg daily are fairly equivalent, and therefore are comparable doses based on the author's clinical experience.

In summary, review of the literature and clinical experience suggest that olanzapine is an atypical antipsychotic with effectiveness for positive and negative symptoms, low risk of EPS, minimal effect on prolactin level at therapeutic doses, and superior tolerability. The insignificant elevation of prolactin level is a distinct advantage over traditional antipsychotics and risperidone. Therefore olanzapine has the potential to become the general purpose first-line antipsychotic of choice among the antipsychotic medications available currently.

Summary of Advantages and Disadvantages of Olanzapine (Zyprexa)

Advantages

- Effective for positive and negative symptoms
- Very low incidence of acute EPS at therapeutic dosage range (dose dependent)

- Probable low risk of tardive dyskinesia (too early to be conclusive)
- Does not elevate prolactin level significantly
- Generally well tolerated
- Once-a-day dosing improves compliance
- Patients can generally be started at an optimal therapeutic dose of 10 mg at bedtime
- Low incidence of sexual dysfunction
- Potential significant long-term cost savings due to decreased illness-related direct and indirect costs

Disadvantages

- Drowsiness, dizziness, dry mouth, and weight gain can be initial side effects (appetite increase can be persistent in some)
- Mild EPS possible at the higher dosage range
- High cost
- Tablets are unscored, making it less convenient to divide
- Parenteral and liquid forms not available as of this writing
- Can occasionally precipitate mania, requiring discontinuation

SERTINDOLE (SERLECT)

Sertindole is a serotonin-dopamine antagonist (SDA) antipsychotic expected to be introduced in the United States in early 1997. It will be available as 4 mg, 8 mg, 20 mg, and 24 mg capsules. Its half-life is three days. Plasma-protein binding is 99.3 percent. Sertindole is effective for both positive and negative symptoms of schizophrenia with virtually no extrapyramidal symptoms in the recommended dosage range. The risk of tardive dyskinesia is therefore expected to be very low; however, chronic exposure to sertindole is necessary to confirm this expectation. There are no significant anticholinergic or sedating effects. Like clozapine, it does not elevate prolactin level. It is generally well tolerated by patients.

Its virtual lack of EPS, efficacy for treating both positive and negative symptoms, lack of elevation of prolactin level, and excellent tolerability should make it one of the front-line general purpose antipsychotics of choice, with clear-cut superiority over the traditional antipsychotics. Sertindole is comparable to olanzapine, though olanzapine has an EPS risk that is slightly greater than that of sertindole. Sertindole compares favorably to risperidone, which causes sustained elevation of prolactin level. Its efficacy in the treatment of treatment-refractory schizophrenia has not been evaluated.

Sertindole can, however, cause mild asymptomatic prolongation of QT interval in approximately 1 percent of patients. There was no episode of torsades de pointes reported among sertindole-treated patients during extensive premarketing clinical trials. It should be mentioned that other antipsychotics, including thioridazine, risperidone, and clozapine, as well as nonpsychiatric drugs such as terfanadine, astemizole, and cisapride, can also cause mild prolongation of QT interval. Patients who may be at risk for prolongation of QT interval are the elderly, patients with bradycardia, preexisting cardiac conduction defects and congestive heart failure, patients taking TCAs or antiarrhythmic agents, and patients taking medications that inhibit the metabolism of sertindole and thus increase its plasma concentration. Fluoxetine and paroxetine are examples among common psychiatric medications that can interact with sertindole in this manner. A 25 to 50 percent reduction in sertindole dose is recommended for patients taking fluoxetine and paroxetine, whereas a 25 to 50 percent sertindole dose increase may be necessary for patients taking carbamazepine or phenytoin. It is recommended that patients be started on a dose of 4 mg daily with 4 mg increments every two to four days as tolerated up to a maximum dose of 24 mg, with a major portion given as a bedtime dose. The effective dosage range in the majority of patients is 12 to 24 mg daily. The gradual titration of dosage to reach the therapeutic dose is to minimize tachycardia and dizziness, which can be initial side effects that typically subside within two to three days of a dosage increase. However, the need for gradual dosage titration makes sertindole unsuitable for controlling acute psychosis unless benzodiazepines and/or other antipsychotics are used adjunctively until sertindole dose can be titrated to a therapeutic range. Lack of sedation and anticholinergic effects are likely to facilitate patient acceptance and tolerability.

Decreased ejaculatory volume can be an initial side effect that tends to improve gradually as the patient continues taking the medication. Decrease in libido, erectile or orgasmic impairment, and retrograde ejaculation have not been reported at an incidence greater than that for placebo. Other side effects include nasal congestion, nausea, rhinitis, postural hypotension, peripheral edema, tachycardia, dizziness, and mild weight gain. Tolerance develops to most of these side effects. Sertindole should be used cautiously with drugs that prolong QT interval (e.g., terfanadine and astemizole) or with drugs that inhibit sertindole metabolism (itraconazole, quinidine, and ketoconazole). Those patients who are at risk for QT prolongation may need EKG monitoring after the dosage titration is completed or after each dosage increment above 12 mg per day, if the physician decides to start sertindole in such a patient. It is also prudent to monitor pulse and blood pressure during the dosage titration period. Routine EKG monitoring is not needed for patients not at risk for QT prolongation. The dosage titration should be slow in the elderly who may be at greater risk for adverse cardiovascular events. If the patient is off sertindole for more than one week, dose retitration may be necessary to arrive at a therapeutic dose. Sertindole metabolism may be enhanced in patients taking carbamazepine or phenytoin.

The dosage should be reduced in the elderly and in patients who have hepatic impairment. Renal patients or patients on hemodialysis may not need dosage adjustment. No correlation has been established between sertindole plasma concentration and efficacy.

Sertindole Dosage Guidelines

- Conditions associated with mild psychotic symptoms such as paranoid, schizotypal and schizoid features, and dementia might respond to doses in the range of 4 to 8 mg daily
- Conditions with moderate psychotic symptoms such as delusional disorders, psychotic symptoms associated with affective disorders, schizoaffective disorders, and bipolar disorder might respond to a dosage range of 8 to 16 mg daily
- Conditions characterized by severe psychotic symptoms such as the schizophrenias and severe schizoaffective disorders might respond to doses in the range of 12 to 24 mg daily

Adjunctive Medications

Psychotropic medications that inhibit or induce hepatic enzymes CYP2D6 and CYP3A could affect the plasma level of sertindole.

Fluoxetine and paroxetine can inhibit sertindole metabolism, necessitating a dose reduction of sertindole. Carbamazepine can induce sertindole metabolism and therefore sertindole dose increase may be necessary. However, most psychotropic medications can be coadministered with sertindole in a combination treatment if necessary, provided dosage adjustment is made to accommodate hepatic enzyme inhibition and induction. In most instances of combination treatment, if fairly low doses of adjunctive medications or low to medium dose range of the primary medications are employed, drug interaction problems due to hepatic enzyme induction and inhibition, and free-plasma drug level variability due to plasma-protein binding effects are usually not of practical clinical concern.

Switching to Sertindole

The general approach is not to switch if the patient is doing well on clozapine, olanzapine, or risperidone. Review the switching guidelines with reference to olanzapine for general clinical principles which should be applicable to sertindole also. However, if the existing antipsychotic has the potential to prolong QT interval, initiation of sertindole titration may have to wait until the patient stops taking the existing antipsychotic, in order to minimize possible additive effects on QT interval. If agitation emerges during the transition period, benzodiazepines may provide control of symptoms without increased cardiovascular risk. A unique requirement of sertindole initiation is the need for gradual dosage titration to reach a therapeutic dose, similar to clozapine initiation, but different from risperidone initiation, which affords a fairly rapid titration, and olanzapine therapy, which can be initiated at the therapeutic dose. Sertindole requires a starting dose of 4 mg per day with a 4 mg increment every two to four days as tolerated to arrive at the therapeutic dose. For instance, it will take approximately ten days to reach a therapeutic sertindole dose of 16 mg. The existing antipsychotic may be gradually tapered off over a ten-day period concurrent with the sertindole titration period. Clozapine taper, however, should ideally be completed slowly, over a 10- to 20-day period to minimize the chance of emergence of clozapine withdrawal symptoms. Again, refer to the section on olanzapine for clinical guidelines that are also applicable to sertindole.

To summarize, sertindole is an atypical antipsychotic with effectiveness for positive and negative symptoms, virtually no risk of extrapyramidal symptoms at therapeutic doses, and no effect on prolactin level. If clinical experience with large numbers of patients confirms the expectation that the prolongation of QT interval is of no clinical significance in terms of patient morbidity, sertindole would be one of the highly useful antipsychotics due to its many advantages and relatively minor disadvantages. Price information was not available at the time of this writing.

Summary of Advantages and Disadvantages of Sertindole

Advantages

- Effective for positive and negative symptoms
- Virtual absence of EPS at therapeutic dose range (equal to placebo)
- Very low risk of tardive dyskinesia (too early to be conclusive)
- No significant anticholinergic or sedating effects
- Does not elevate prolactin level
- Does not affect libido or sexual performance (reduced ejaculatory volume frequently improves over time)
- Long half-life enables once-a-day dosing, enhancing compliance
- Generally well tolerated
- Improved efficacy and tolerability should decrease relapses and rehospitalizations
- Potential significant long-term cost savings due to decreased illness-related direct and indirect costs
- Possible medication cost savings due to expected availability of convenient 20 and 24 mg capsules

Disadvantages

- Mild prolongation of the QT interval (routine EKG screening/ monitoring is not recommended. However, EKG monitoring may be considered in susceptible patients, e.g., the elderly, patient with congestive heart failure, bradycardia and left ven-

tricular hypertrophy, and patients taking TCAs or antiarrhythmia agents.); rare incidence of sudden death reported during clinical trials has not been attributed to arrhythmia induced by sertindole
- Need for gradual upward titration of dose (due to tachycardia and hypotension if started on a higher initial dose, or if dose is rapidly increased)
- Retitration may be needed if patients are off sertindole for more than one week
- Capsule form makes it inconvenient to divide
- Parenteral and liquid forms not available currently
- Medication cost expected to be high

(Price information unavailable at the time of this writing.)

Appendix A

Alphabetical Listing of Drugs by Generic Names, with U.S. Brand Names

Generic Name	Brand Name
alprazolam	Xanax
amantadine	Symmetrel
amitriptyline	Elavil, Endep
amitriptyline + perphenazine	Triavil, Etrafon
amitriptyline + chlordiazepoxide	Limbitrol
amoxapine	Asendin
atenolol	Tenormin
benztropine	Cogentin
biperiden	Akineton
bromocriptine	Parlodel
bupropion	Wellbutrin
buspirone	BuSpar
carbamazepine	Tegretol
chloral hydrate	Noctec
chlordiazepoxide	Librium
chlordiazepoxide + amitriptyline	Limbitrol
chlorpromazine	Thorazine
chlorprothixene	Taractan

Generic Name	Brand Name
clomipramine	Anafranil
clonazepam	Klonopin
clonidine	Catapres
clorazepate	Tranxene
clozapine	Clozaril
cyproheptadine	Periactin
dantrolene	Dantrium
desipramine	Norpramin, Pertofrane
dextroamphetamine	Dexedrine
diazepam	Valium
diphenhydramine	Benadryl
disulfiram	Antabuse
divalproex sodium	Depakote, Depakote Sprinkle
doxepin	Sinequan, Adapin
estazolam	Prosom
fenfluramine	Pondimin
fluoxetine	Prozac
fluphenazine	Prolixin, Permitil
flurazepam	Dalmane
fluvoxamine	Luvox
gabapentin	Neurontin
guanfacine	Tenex
haloperidol	Haldol
hydroxyzine	Vistaril, Atarax
imipramine	Tofranil, Janimine
isocarboxazid	Marplan (discontinued)
lamotrigine	Lamictal

Generic Name	Brand Name
levothyroxine (T4)	Synthroid, Levoxine
liothyronine (T3)	Cytomel
lithium	Eskalith, Lithobid, Lithonate, Cibalith
lorazepam	Ativan
loxapine	Loxitane
maprotiline	Ludiomil
mesoridazine	Serentil
methylphenidate	Ritalin
mirtazapine	Remeron
molindone	Moban
naltrexone	Revia, Trexan
nefazodone	Serzone
nifedipine	Procardia
nortriptyline	Pamelor, Aventyl
olanzapine	Zyprexa
oxazepam	Serax
paroxetine	Paxil
pemoline	Cylert
perphenazine	Trilafon
perphenazine + amitriptyline	Triavil, Etrafon
phenelzine	Nardil
phenobarbital	Luminal
pindolol	Visken
prazepam	Centrax
procyclidine	Kemadrin
propranolol	Inderal

Generic Name	Brand Name
protriptyline	Vivactil
quazepam	Doral
risperidone	Risperdal
sertindole	Serlect
sertraline	Zoloft
sodium divalproex	Depakote
sodium valproate	Depakene
temazepam	Restoril
thioridazine	Mellaril
thiothixene	Navane
tranylcypromine	Parnate
trazodone	Desyrel
triazolam	Halcion
trifluoperazine	Stelazine
trihexyphenidyl	Artane
trimipramine	Surmontil
valproate	Depakene
valproic acid	Depakene
venlafaxine	Effexor
verapamil	Calan, Isoptin
yohimbine	Yocon
zolpidem	Ambien

Appendix B

Alphabetical Listing of Drugs by U.S. Brand Names, with Generic Names

Brand Name	Generic Name
Adapin	doxepin
Akineton	biperiden
Ambien	zolpidem
Anafranil	clomipramine
Antabuse	disulfiram
Artane	trihexyphenidyl
Asendin	amoxapine
Atarax	hydroxyzine
Ativan	lorazepam
Aventyl	nortriptyline
Benadryl	diphenhydramine
BuSpar	buspirone
Calan	verapamil
Catapres	clonidine
Centrax	prazepam
Cibalith-s	lithium citrate (syrup)
Clozaril	clozapine
Cogentin	benztropine

Brand Name	Generic Name
Cylert	pemoline
Cytomel	liothyronine (T3)
Dalmane	flurazepam
Dantrium	dantrolene
Depakene	valproate, valproic acid, sodium valproate
Depakote	divalproex sodium, sodium divalproex
Depakote Sprinkle	divalproex sodium, sodium divalproex
Desyrel	trazodone
Dexedrine	dextroamphetamine
Doral	quazepam
Effexor	venlafaxine
Elavil	amitriptyline
Endep	amitriptyline
Eskalith	lithium
Etrafon	perphenazine + amitriptyline
Halcion	triazolam
Haldol	haloperidol
Inderal	propranolol
Isoptin	verapamil
Janimine	imipramine
Kemadrin	procyclidine
Klonopin	clonazepam
Lamictal	lamotrigine
Levoxine	levothyroxine (T4)
Librium	chlordiazepoxide

Brand Name	Generic Name
Limbitrol	chlordiazepoxide + amitriptyline
Lithobid	lithium
Lithonate	lithium
Lithotabs	lithium
Loxitane	loxapine
Ludiomil	maprotiline
Luminal	phenobarbital
Luvox	fluvoxamine
Marplan	isocarboxazid (discontinued)
Mellaril	thioridazine
Moban	molindone
Nardil	phenelzine
Navane	thiothixene
Neurontin	gabapentin
Noctec	chloral hydrate
Norpramin	desipramine
Pamelor	nortriptyline
Parlodel	bromocriptine
Parnate	tranylcypromine
Paxil	paroxetine
Periactin	cyproheptadine
Permitil	fluphenazine
Pertofrane	desipramine
Pondimin	fenfluramine
Procardia	nifedipine
Prolixin	fluphenazine
ProSom	estazolam

Brand Name	Generic Name
Prozac	fluoxetine
Remeron	mirtazapine
Restoril	temazepam
Revia	naltrexone
Risperdal	risperidone
Ritalin	methylphenidate
Serax	oxazepam
Serentil	mesoridazine
Serlect	sertindole
Serzone	nefazodone
Sinequan	doxepin
Stelazine	trifluoperazine
Surmontil	trimipramine
Symmetrel	amantadine
Synthroid	levothyroxine (T4)
Taractan	chlorprothixene
Tegretol	carbamazepine
Tenex	guanfacine
Tenormin	atenolol
Thorazine	chlorpromazine
Tofranil	imipramine
Tranxene	clorazepate
Trexan	naltrexone
Triavil	perphenazine + amitriptyline
Trilafon	perphenazine
Valium	diazepam
Visken	pindolol

Brand Name	Generic Name
Vistaril	hydroxyzine
Vivactil	protriptyline
Wellbutrin	bupropion
Xanax	alprazolam
Yocon	yohimbine
Zoloft	sertraline
Zypexa	olanzapine

Appendix C

Alphabetical Listing of Abbreviations

AC	before meals
ADD	attention deficit disorder
ADHD	attention deficit hyperactivity disorder
BID	twice a day
CBC	complete blood count
DSM	*Diagnostic and Statistical Manual of Mental Disorders*
ECG	electrocardiogram
ECT	electroconvulsive therapy
EKG	electrocardiogram
EPS	extrapyramidal symptoms
GAD	generalized anxiety disorder
GI	gastrointestinal
HS	at night; at bedtime
IM	intramuscular
IV	intravenous
MAO	monoamine oxidase
MAOI	monoamine oxidase inhibitor
mcg	microgram
mcl	microliter
mEq/L	milliequivalent per liter

mg	milligram
ng	nanogram
NMS	neuroleptic malignant syndrome
OCD	obsessive-compulsive disorder
OTC	over the counter
PC	after meals
po	by mouth
PRN	as needed
PTSD	post-traumatic stress disorder
QD	daily, every day
QOD	every other day
Qhs	every night
QID	four times a day
SSRI	selective serotonin reuptake inhibitor
TCA	tricyclic antidepressant
TD	tardive dyskinesia
TID	three times a day
TSH	thyroid stimulating hormone
WBC	white blood cell count

Bibliography

American Medical Association. (1994). *Drug Evaluations Annual.* Washington, DC.

American Psychiatric Association. (1994). *Diagnostic and Statistical Manual of Mental Disorders,* Fourth Edition. Washington, DC.

American Society of Hospital Pharmacists. (1994). *Drug Information 1994.* Bethesda, MD.

Appleton, W. S. (1988). *Practical Clinical Psychopharmacology, Third Edition.* Baltimore, MD: Williams and Wilkins.

Ayd, F. J. (1994). Clozapine. 1994: Clinical Considerations. *International Drug Therapy Newsletter* 29 (May/June): 21-28.

Balon, R., Yeragani, V. K., Pohl, R., and Ramesh, C. (1993). Sexual dysfunction during antidepressant treatment. *Journal of Clinical Psychiatry* 54: 209-212.

Beasley, C. M., Tollefson, G., Tran, P., Satterlee, W., Sanger, T., Hamilton, S., and the Olanzapine Study Group. (1996). Olanzapine versus placebo and haloperidol. *Neuropsychopharmacology,* 14(2): 83-85.

Blier, P. and Bergeron, R. (1995). Effectiveness of Pindolol with Selected Antidepressant Drugs in the Treatment of Major Depression. *Journal of Clinical Psychopharmacology* 15 (June): 217-222.

Bodkin, J. A., Cohen, B. M., Salomon, M. S., Cannon, S. E., Zornberg, G. L., and Cole, J. O. (1996). Treatment of negative symptoms in schizophrenia and schizoaffective disorder by selegiline augmentation of antipsychotic medication. *Journal of Nervous and Mental Disease* 184: 295-301.

Borison, R. L. (1995). Clinical efficacy of serotonin-dopamine antagonists relative to classic neuroleptics. *Journal of Clinical Psychopharmacology* 15(1) suppl. 1: 24S-29S.

Brenner, J. (1995). Double-blind comparison of org 3770, amitriptyline, and placebo in major depression. *Journal of Clinical Psychiatry* 56: 519-525.
Breier, A., Buchanan, R. W., Kirkpatrick, B., Davis, O., Irish, D., Summerfelt, A., and Carpenter, W. (1994). Effects of clozapine on positive and negative symptoms in outpatients with schizophrenia. *American Journal of Psychiatry* 151: 20-26.
Ciraulo, D. A. and Shader, R. I. (1991). *Clinical Manual of Chemical Dependence*. Washington, DC: American Psychiatric Press, Inc.
Compendium Publications Group. (1994) *Physicians' Compendium of Drug Therapy*. Secaucus, NJ.
Coffey, C. E. (1993). *The Clinical Science of Electroconvulsive Therapy*. Washington, DC: American Psychiatric Press, Inc.
DeVane, C. L. (1994). Pharmacogenetics and drug metabolism of newer antidepressant agents. *Journal of Clinical Psychiatry* 55: 38-45.
Guttmacher, L. B. (1988). *Somatic Therapies in Psychiatry*. Washington, DC: American Psychiatric Press, Inc.
Hyman, S. E., Arana, G. W., and Rosenbaum, J. F. (1995). *Handbook of Psychiatric Drug Therapy*. Third Edition. Boston, MA: Little, Brown.
Janicak, P. G., Davis, J. M., Preskorn, S. H., and Ayd, F. J. Jr. (1993). *Principles and Practice of Psychopharmacotherapy*. Baltimore, MD: Williams & Wilkins.
Joseph, S. (1997). *Symptom-Focused Psychiatric Drug Therapy for Managed Care, With 100 Clinical Cases*. Binghamton, NY: The Haworth Press.
Kane, J. M., Honigfeld, G., Singer, J., and Meltzer, H. (1988). Clozapine for the treatment-resistant schizophrenic: A double-blind comparison with chlorpromazine. *Archives of General Psychiatry* 45: 789-796.
Kaplan, H. I. and Sadeck, B. J. (Editors). (1989). *Comprehensive Textbook of Psychiatry/V, Fifth Edition*. Baltimore, MD: Williams & Wilkins.
Kehoe, W. A. and Schorr, R. B. (1996). Focus on mirtazapine: A new antidepressant with noradrenergic and specific serotonergic activity. *Formulary* 31: 455-469.

Lieberman, J. A., Kane, J. M., and Johns, P. A. (1989). Clozapine: Guidelines for clinical management. *Journal of Clinical Psychiatry* 50: 329-338.

Marder, S. R. and Meibach, R. C. (1994). Risperidone in the treatment of schizophrenia. *American Journal of Psychiatry* 151: 825-835.

Maxmen, J. S. (1991). *Psychotropic Drugs–Fast Facts.* New York: W. W. Norton & Company.

McEroy, S. L., Dessain, E. R., Pope, H. G., Cole, J., Keck, P., Frankenberg, F., Aizley, H., and O'Brien, S. (1991). Clozapine in the treatment of psychotic mood disorder, schizoaffective disorder, and schizophrenia. *Journal of Clinical Psychiatry* 52: 411-414.

Meltzer, H. Y. (editor). (1992). *Novel antipsychotic drugs.* New York: Raven Press.

Meltzer, H. Y. (1994). An overview of the mechanism of action of clozapine. *Journal of Clinical Psychiatry* 55, suppl. B: 46-52.

Meltzer, H. Y. and Fibiger, H. C. (1996). Olanzapine: A new antipsychotic drug. *Neuropsychopharmacology* 14(2): 83-85.

Physicians' Desk Reference. (1996). Montvale, NJ: Medical Economics Company.

Richelson, E. (1994). Preclinical pharmacology of antipsychotic drugs: Relationship to efficacy and side effects. *Journal of Clinical Psychiatry* Monograph 12(2):17-20.

Rosse, R. B., Giese, A. A., Deutsch, S. I., and Morihisa, J. M. (1989). *Laboratory Diagnostic Testing in Psychiatry.* Washington, DC: American Psychiatric Press, Inc.

Roth, A. S., Ostroff, R. B., and Hoffman, R. E. (1996). Naltrexone as a treatment for repetitive self-injurious behavior: An open-label trial. *Journal of Clinical Psychiatry,* 57: 233-237.

Sandoz Pharmaceutical Corporation. (1993). *Clozaril–Management of Adverse Events.* East Hanover, NJ.

Sandoz Pharmaceutical Corporation. (1994). *Standards of Care in Schizophrenia.* East Hanover, NJ.

Sandoz Pharmaceutical Corporation. (1995). *Clozaril Treatment Trends.* East Hanover, NJ.

Schatzberg, A. F. and Nemeroff, C. B. (Editors). (1995). *Textbook of Psychopharmacology.* Washington, DC: American Psychiatric Press, Inc.

Schatzberg, A. F. and Cole, J. O. (1991). *Manual of Clinical Psychopharmacology.* Washington, DC: American Psychiatric Press, Inc.

Tollefson, G. D. (1994). Olanzapine: A novel antipsychotic with a broad spectrum profile. *Neuropsychopharmacology* 10, suppl. 3: 805.

Van Kammen, D. P., McEvoy, J. P., Targum, S. D., Kardatzke, D., Sebree, T., and the Sertindole Study Group. (1996). A randomized, controlled, dose-ranging trial of sertindole in patients with schizophrenia. *Journal of Clinical Psychopharmacology* 124: 168-175.

Index

ADD/ADHD. *See* Attention-deficit/ hyperactivity disorder
Adjustment disorder
  with anxiety, 66
  with depressed mood, 66,168
Admission, involuntary, 42-44
Adolescent(s), interviewing, 8
Agranulocytosis, clozapine induced, 221-222,226,229
Alcohol
  abuse/dependence, 52,138,163, 179
  behavioral effects of, 5-6
Alprazolam, 147,152,155,165,171
Ambien. *See* Zolpidem
Anafranil. *See* Clomipramine
Antidepressants, 33-34
Antipsychotics, 33
  atypical, 209-251
Antisocial personality disorder, 5-6, 75-85
  clinical cases, 79-85
  DSM-IV criteria for, 75
  pharmacotherapy of, 77-79
  symptom correlates of, 76
Ativan. *See* Lorazepam
Attention-deficit disorder (ADD), 56,82,84,135
Attention-deficit hyperactivity disorder (ADHD), 77,187
Avoidant personality disorder, 143, 147
  clinical case, 146-148
  DSM-IV criteria for, 143
  pharmacotherapy of, 144-146
  symptom correlates of, 144

Benadryl. *See* Diphenhydramine
Benzodiazepines, for paranoid personality disorder, 29-30
Benztropine, 65,105
Bipolar disorder, NOS, 71,100,108, 110,112,139,179
Borderline personality disorder, 87, 96,98,100,101,102,105,108, 110,112,114,120
  clinical cases, 96-121
  DSM-IV criteria for, 87
  pharmacotherapy of, 88-96
  symptom correlates of, 89
Brain
  behavior and, 5
  injury, 4
Bupropion, 56,82,100,120,128,153, 185-188
  advantages of, 187
  cost data, 186
  disadvantages of, 188
  dosage and administration, 185-187
  side effects, 185-187
Bupropion SR, 188-190
  advantages of, 189
  disadvantages of, 190
  dosage and administration, 188-189
  side effects, 188-189

Cannabis dependence, 100,135
Carbamazepine, 41,179
Cases. *See specific personality disorders*
Chlordiazepoxide, 138
Chlorpromazine, 105
Clomipramine, 41,66,72,105,163, 206
  advantages, 207

Clomipramine *(continued)*
disadvantages, 207
dosage and administration, 206-207
side effects, 206-207
Clonazepam, 96,110,141,169
Clonidine, 112
Clozapine, 99,101,102,108,115,212
advantages, 236
agranulocytosis caused by, 221,228
community mental health centers (CMHCs) and, 238-239
cost data, 223
disadvantages, 237
dosage and administration, 213-235
side effects and their management, 227,230-232
Clozaril. *See* Clozapine
Cogentin. *See* Benztropine
Cognitive-behavioral therapy, 49,160
Community mental health centers, clozapine use in, 238-239
Conduct disorder, 84, 112
clinical case, 84-85
Cyclothymia, 108

Delirium, 6
Depakene. *See* Valproic acid
Dapakote. *See* Valproate
Dependent personality disorder, 149,152-153,155-156
clinical cases, 151-156
DSM-IV criteria for, 149
pharmacotherapy of, 150-151
symptom correlates of, 150
Depression
in avoidant personality disorder, 144
in borderline personality disorder, 89,91
in dependent personality disorder, 150
Desyrel. *See* Trazodone
Dexedrine. *See* Dextroamphetamine
Dextroamphetamine, 84
Diazepam, 114
Diphenhydramine, 100
Divalproex sodium. *See* Valproate
Dose-response curve, 17
Doxepin, 166
Dysthymia, 52,56,82,84,96,141,153, 156,171,179

Effexor. *See* Venlafaxine
Eskalith. *See* Lithium
Evolution, in psychiatric drug therapy, 23

Fluoxetine, 36,51,56,62,68,69,71,80, 82,101,108,112,167,168,170, 174,179,190-192
advantages of, 191
cost data, 192
disadvantages of, 191-192
dosage and administration, 190-191
side effects, 191
Fluvoxamine, 135,171,199-201
advantages, 200
cost data, 200
disadvantages, 201
dosage and administration, 199-200
side effects, 200

Gabapentin, 226
Generalized anxiety disorder, 169

Haldol. *See* Haloperidol
Haloperidol, 99
Histrionic personality disorder, 122, 128
clinical case, 127-129
DSM-IV criteria for, 123

Histrionic personality disorder
(continued)
pharmacotherapy of, 125-127
symptom correlates of, 124
Hospitalization, for clozapine
initiation, 227
Hypomania, 77

Ideas of reference, 26,27
Imipramine, 147
Inderal. *See* Propranolol
Involuntary treatment, 43,44

Kleptomania, 101
Klonopin. *See* Clonazepam

Lamotrigine, 226
Librium. *See* Chlordiazepoxide
Lithium, 65,71,102,108,110,120,
135,139
Lithobid. *See* Lithium
Lorazepam, 72,73,99

Major depressive disorder, 96,98,
101,120,138,152,153,155,
156,166,174
Managed care, xvi
Mania and pseudomania,
distinguishing features, 126
MAOI(s). *See* Monoamine oxidase
inhibitors
Mellaril. *See* Thioridazine
Mesoridazine, 72
Methylphenidate, 135
Mirtazapine, 203
advantages, 205
cost data, 205
disadvantages, 205
dosage and administration,
204-205
side effects, 204
Monoamine oxidase inhibitors,
33,47,48,49,52,58,62,91,93,
98,102,117,120,144,145,146,
150,162,168,187,191,192,
194,195,196,197,199,202,
203,205,206,220,241,263
Multiple personality disorder, 105

Naltrexone, 138,207-208
Narcissistic personality disorder,
131,135,138,139,141
clinical cases, 135-142
DSM-IV criteria for, 131
pharmacotherapy of, 132-135
symptom correlates of, 133
Nefazodone, 139,201
advantages, 203
cost data, 202
disadvantages, 203
dosage and administration,
201-203
side effects, 202
Neurontin. *See* Gabapentin
Nicotine, 6
Noncompliance, 116
Normalcy-psychosis continuum, 60
Nortriptyline, 120

Obsessive-compulsive disorder, 54,
65,101,105
Obsessive-compulsive personality
disorder, 157,163,165,166,
167,168,169,170,171
clinical cases, 162-172
DSM-IV criteria for, 157
pharmacotherapy of, 158-162
symptom correlates of, 159
Olanzapine, 239
advantages, 245
cost data, 245
disadvantages, 246
dosage and administration,
239-245

Olanzapine *(continued)*
side effects, 240
switching schedule, 242-244

Pamelor. *See* Nortriptyline
Panic disorder, 147,152,171
Paranoid personality disorder
clinical cases, 35-44
DSM-IV criteria for, 25
pharmacotherapy of, 27-35
symptom correlates of, 26
Parkinsonism, 215
Paroxetine, 39,52,54,65,84,102,114,
138,141,147,152,156,165,
166,169,194-196
advantages, 196
cost data, 195
disadvantages, 196
dosage and administration,
194-195
side effects, 194
Paxil. *See* Paroxetine
Pedophilia, 54
Perphenazine, 27,33,36,109,179,
180,181,253,255,258,260
Personality change due to a general
medical condition, 175,179
clinical case, 178
DSM-IV criteria for, 176
pharmacotherapy of, 177-178
subtypes of, 177
Personality disorder(s). *See specific disorders*
cluster A, 14
cluster B, 14
cluster C, 14
Personality disorder, NOS, 173-174
clinical case, 173-184
DSM-IV criteria for, 173
pharmacotherapy of, 173
Pharmacotherapy, compared to
psychotherapy, 9-12
Polypharmacy, rational, 23
Polysubstance abuse, 112
Post-traumatic stress disorder, 88,91
Propranolol, 65,96,108
Prozac. *See* Fluoxetine
Pseudomania, 125,126
compared to mania, 126
Psychiatric disorder, age of onset,
15-16
Psychiatric evaluation, 7
Psychoanalysis, 3-4
Psychotherapy, 9-12

Quality of life, clozapine therapy
and, 237

Rapport, in interview, 8
Remeron. *See* Mirtazapine
Restoril. *See* Temazepam
Risperdal. *See* Risperidone
Risperidone, 36,39,51,52,54,56,62,
65,66,68,69,71,73,80,96,100,
105,108,110,114,128,135,
138,139,141,155,156,174,
209
advantages, 212
cost data, 211
disadvantages, 212
dosage and administration,
209-211
side effects, 209-211
Ritalin. *See* Methylphenidate

Schizoaffective disorder, 65,80,98,
102,105,114
Schizoid personality disorder, 45,52,
54,56
clinical cases, 50-56
DSM-IV criteria for, 45
pharmacotherapy of, 47-50
symptom correlates of, 46
Schizophrenia, 209-251
Schizotypal personality disorder,
57,62,65,67,69,70,72,73
clinical cases, 62-74

Schizotypal personality disorder
(continued)
DSM-IV criteria for, 57
pharmacotherapy of, 58-62
symptom correlates of, 59
Seizure
bupropion and, 185,190
clomipramine and, 206-207
clozapine related, 117,226
Self-mutilation
in borderline personality disorder, 91
naltrexone for, 208
Serlect. *See* Sertindole
Sertindole, 246
advantages, 250
disadvantages, 250
dosage and administration, 246-249
side effects, 246-249
Sertraline, 73,108,192-194
advantages, 193
cost data, 193
disadvantages, 194
dosage and administration, 192-193
side effects, 192-193
Serzone. *See* Nefazodone
Simple deteriorative disorder, 51
Sinequan. *See* Doxepin
Sleep-walking disorder, 163
Social phobia, 144,145
Social skills training, 49
Social withdrawal in schizoid personality disorder, 46-47
Stelazine. *See* Trifluoperazine
Stimulant(s), 91,125
Suicidal behavior, management of, 94-96

Tardive dyskinesia, 212,237,242,250
Tegretol. *See* Carbamazepine
Temazepam, 62,105,156,166,168
Thioridazine, 27,34,56,101,102,103, 114,211,234,243,247,256,259
Thorazine. *See* Chlorpromazine
Tofranil. *See* Imipramine
Trazodone, 52,96,100,105,108,110, 120,138,153,156,168
Trexan. *See* Naltrexone
Triavil (perphenazine and amitriptyline), 112, 169,179
Trilafon. *See* Perphenazine
Trifluoperazine, 41

Utilization review, 236

Valium. *See* Diazepam
Valproate, 110,112,115,141
Valproic acid. *See* Valproate
Venlafaxine, 96,98,153,155,196-199
advantages, 198
cost data, 198
disadvantages, 199
dosage and administration, 196-198
side effects, 197

Wellbutrin. *See* Bupropion
Wellbutrin SR. *See* Bupropion SR

Xanax. *See* Alprazolam

Zoloft. *See* Sertraline
Zolpidem, 39,68,174
Zyprexa. *See* Olanzapine

For Product Safety Concerns and Information please contact our EU representative GPSR@taylorandfrancis.com Taylor & Francis Verlag GmbH, Kaufingerstraße 24, 80331 München, Germany

Batch number: 10725802

Printed by Printforce, the Netherlands